Health and Long Life
The Chinese Way

Three Pines Press
Cambridge, Mass.

Health
and
Long Life

The Chinese Way

by

Livia Kohn

in cooperation with Stephen Jackowicz

Three Pines Press
303 Cambridge Street, #410071
Cambridge, MA 02141
www.threepinespress.com

9 8 7 6 5 4 3 2 1

First Edition, 2005
Printed in the United States of America
⊗ This edition is printed on acid-free paper that meets
the American National Standard Institute Z39.48 Standard.
Distributed in the United States by Three Pines Press.

Library of Congress Cataloging-in-Publication Data

Kohn, Livia, 1956-
   Health and long life the Chinese way / by Livia Kohn in cooperation
with Stephen Jackowicz.-- 1st ed.
      p. cm.
   Includes bibliographical references and index.
   ISBN 1-931483-03-5 (alk. paper)
   1. Medicine, Chinese. 2. Health. 3. Longevity. I. Title.
   R601.K64 2005
   613--dc22
                              2005002026

Contents

List of Illustrations

Dynastic Chart

B.C.E.	Shang	1766-1122
	Western Zhou	1122-770
	Eastern Zhou	770-221
	Qin	221-206
	Former Han	206-6
C.E.	Later Han	23-220
	Three Kingdoms	220-265
	Western Jin	265-317
	Eastern Jin	317-420
	Six Dynasties	420-589
	Sui	589-618
	Tang	618-907
	Five Dynasties	907-960
	Northern Song	960-1126
	Southern Song	1126-1260
	Mongol-Yuan	1260-1368
	Ming	1368-1644
	Manchu-Qing	1644-1911
	Republic (Taiwan)	1911-
	People's Republic	1949-

Acknowledgments

This book grew from a class on Chinese medicine and religious healing techniques that I have taught at Boston University since 1989. Developed from a background of Daoist studies and the examination of Chinese longevity techniques, the class is a lecture with some student presentations that covers both the basic worldview and the varying practices of East Asian health traditions. As the course unfolded and was modified over the years, it has become more encompassing yet simpler in its presentation, enhancing the overall understanding of Chinese health and longevity practices.

This book follows the structure of the class. Its central purpose is to give a basic overview of East Asian medical and spiritual techniques while allowing readers to delve further into specific areas of interest. As a secondary goal, it also takes on the question of where Chinese healing is located in relation to both the contemporary Western understanding of body and mind and the traditional doctrines and practices of the Daoist religion. It asks, therefore, how Chinese health techniques work, how their worldview can be understood in modern terms, and how they are related to religious Daoism.

With regard to the latter, it is common to see the worldview of yin-yang and the five phases as Daoist, when both form in fact an aspect of Chinese cosmology that is ubiquitous in the culture and cannot be linked with one specific tradition. On the other hand, Daoist techniques of breathing and meditation, although used in health practice, have a deep spiritual dimension and are often seen only in their medical role. The interaction of the traditions is multifaceted and complex. Still, it can be said in general that Chinese medicine, the pursuit of long life, and Daoist religious cultivation all form different aspects on the same continuum, follow the same underlying worldview, and apply closely related techniques, though in somewhat different ways and toward different ultimate purposes.

Each chapter in the book begins by presenting core information on the basic worldview and practices of Chinese health and longevity techniques, then examines the problem of their interrelation with modern and traditional models. As a basic overview, the work is well suited to serve as a textbook in classes on Chinese medicine, religion, and culture.

As an analytical volume, it is useful to practitioners who wish to understand the religious and spiritual background of their art. Last but not least, as a primer it is helpful to the general public interested in how the Chinese envisioned health and what methods they use to maintain it into advanced old age.

The book was not created by my efforts alone. I am very much indebted to the students of my class at Boston University who over the years have contributed much to the shaping of the course and the organization of its contents. Beyond that, many friends and colleagues have helped with their insights, suggestions, and criticisms as well as with their books, conference presentations, and lectures. Most importantly, my former student, colleague, and medical adviser Stephen Jackowicz was a staunch cooperator during the entire production. He wrote parts of the introduction and various chapters, notably those on Dao and *qi* (ch. 1), diagnosis (ch. 6), acupuncture (ch. 7), and Chinese medicine in other East Asian countries (ch. 10) — which incidentally appeared separately as a co-authored article in *Oriental Medicine* 13.1 (Jan. 2005) — and has shownunflagging encouragement and support. I am most grateful for his partnership.

The entire manuscript was read and criticized by my dear friends and colleagues Shawn Arthur, Ute Engelhardt, Lonny Jarrett, Michael Leonard, Kate Townsend, Dennis Willmont, and Michael Winn. They all combine a tremendous dedication to practice with a thorough understanding of the tradition and a never-ending inquisitiveness about its spiritual dimensions and historical origins. They have shaped the book in more ways than one. Beyond that, I am especially grateful to Bede Bidlack and Vincent Mitchell, martial arts practitioners extraordinaire and to me both students and teachers. Without them I could not have written the chapter on Taiji quan. Be they all be thanked from the bottom of my heart.

Introduction

For over 2,000 years, the Chinese have been experts at maintaining health and extending longevity. Their methods, documented in ancient manuscripts, medical textbooks, and self-cultivation manuals, form a multi-layered yet integrated system of personalized health care that is of increasing value in the West as our population ages and technology increases the speed and stresses of our life.

In the past thirty years, since Richard Nixon first went to China and acupuncture became known to the general Western public, Chinese methods of health enhancement have made great inroads in Western societies. There are now thousands of professionally trained acupuncture, herbal, and massage practitioners, joined by an ever increasing number of Fengshui, Taiji quan, and Qigong masters. About three-quarters of the American population report that they have at least tried some form of complementary, often Chinese, health practice, and the overall trend is toward further increase and growing popularity. This is partly due to the rise in the cost of hospitals and HMOs, but more importantly it is in response to the perceived lack of Western biomedicine. As Manfred Porkert already noted in 1988:

> Science has prolonged our lives, but the ideal of health still remains elusive. Numerous "new" diseases have rise to take the place of old ones that doctors have learned to deal with and medical science has thoroughly investigated, and against them Western medicine is powerless—or there is not all that much that can be done. (*Chinese Medicine*, 16)

In addition to AIDS, SARS, and new forms of cancer and the flu which plague modern humanity, more people than ever before suffer from chronic ailments, degenerative conditions, allergies, stress-induced syndromes, or psychosomatic diseases. For example, numerous of Americans are in chronic pain, and two-thirds of all employees suffer from some kind of pain condition. They take over billions of Aspirin every year. Also, over half of the population is overweight or obese, and one-fifth suffers from hypertension. Innumerable people have trouble sleep-

1

ing and continuously take drugs to keep themselves functioning, Many are plagued by anxiety and depression, taking millions of pounds of stimulants, anti-anxiety drugs, and ACE inhibitors every year.

All too often patients see their physicians with a set of symptoms that do not easily yield to standard classifications, receive some remedies that help for a while or to some extent, then are left again with their condition. The patients, tired and ailing, will seek a second opinion, make the rounds of the specialists, but may well end up with a fresh disappointment to add to their original troubles. Often, as John Abramson points out, they are given "expensive drugs when lifestyle changes would be far more effective at protecting health" and have to undergo "tests and consultations that are very unlikely to lead to better outcomes" (*Over-do$ed America*, 53). Even more disturbing, medical errors and iatrogenic diseases are the third leading cause of death in the U.S., undermining what little confidence patients might have left.

It is thus not surprising that patients seek an integrated approach to health, a methodology that takes their whole being, lifestyle, and social situation into account and that promises long-term relief and a high quality of health. Many turn to Chinese modalities, choosing among different techniques offered—from acupuncture, herbs, and massages through Fengshui, diets, gymnastics, and meditations to Qigong and Taiji quan. All part of the greater Chinese health effort, they share the same underlying worldview, expressed in various theoretical concepts: Dao, the fundamental way of the universe that determines all existence; *qi*, the cosmic vital force or energy that pervades life and determines the functioning of the human body and mind; yin-yang, the two complementary aspects of Dao that alternate in their interaction to create the rhythms of nature and the body; and the five phases, the basis of an extensive correspondence system at the root of diagnosis and treatment.

Although expressed in a clear, unambiguous vocabulary, consistent in itself, free from internal contradictions, and applied with sophisticated techniques of observation and diagnosis, the vocabulary and concepts of Chinese health methods are quite alien to Western thinking. To be applied successfully, they require not only patient explanation but the willingness to give up prejudices and preconceptions and immerse oneself in a totally unfamiliar language. Still, opening oneself to this alternative understanding can be very rewarding. It may lead to a completely new way of looking at the body and the world and enlarge one's spectrum of attainable health and personal realization.

It is the first task of this book to present the basic concepts underlying Chinese ways to health and long life in a simple and straightforward manner, placing them into a dynamic internal context and relating them to comparative Western ideas.

Armed with a good grip of the fundamentals, one can then venture to make sense of the many apparently unconnected methods that aim at different dimensions in the pursuit of health. Some, like acupuncture and massages, are administered to the patient by a trained professional and require nothing more than keeping an appointment and resting peacefully on the treatment table. Others, like diets, herbs, Fengshui, and sexual techniques involve methods that the patient can do for himself or herself in interaction with foodstuffs, the environment, and other people. To be effective, these methods need some self-control and a certain degree of discipline. Yet others are forms of meditation and self-cultivation, such as breathing, gymnastics, Taiji quan, Qigong, and meditations. Undertaken by the patient in classes and private practice, they have to be followed over longer periods of time to bring about health and transformation. The book follows the different methods in this order, presenting first clinical, medical therapies, then ways of interactive *qi*-control, and last spiritual ways of self-cultivation.

All these methods have their own role in the larger Chinese health care system. As "to heal" means "to make whole," they all serve to transform human beings from simple discreet entities separate from the outside world into active participants in the triad of heaven, earth, and humanity. Chinese health methods not only cure and vitalize people's bodies and minds, but aim to join them harmoniously with the larger cosmos. Health accordingly does not just mean the absence of illness or symptoms, but is an integrated balance of physical well-being, personal happiness, good fortune, and harmony. Healing is less the direct, objective treatment of diseases than the gentle prodding of the body-mind to remember how to restore itself to perfect function.

Within this larger picture, treatments administered by a trained practitioner include mainly acupuncture and massage, but they are not homogeneous or formally standardized. Rather, in the course of history, they have developed into different forms and schools in China and were also transmitted to Vietnam, Korean, and Japan, where they took on various local modalities. As a result, acupuncture needles vary in length and thickness, methods of insertion are manifold, diagnoses follow different principles, and the points of needling may not be the same. Massages, too, while using the same clinical system as acupuncture, may include greater or lesser degrees of muscular therapy and structural alignments, strong hands-on kneading of tissues or the distant *qi*-emission in a laying-on of hands.

Self-healing methods undertaken in interaction with the outside world and other people, second, range from the systematic guiding of *qi* in one's environment with the help of Fengshui through its regulation through food, diets, and herbs to its enhancement with sexual techniques. Here, too, a variety of schools and applications has grown both in China and through the transmission to other countries, so that, for example, diets can be as diverse as recommending an all-cooked or all-raw regimen, emphasizing the need for starches or insisting on the complete avoidance of grain.

Third, practitioners of self-cultivation can choose from breathing exercises, gymnastics, Qigong, Taiji quan, and various forms of meditation. These techniques reach far into the religious dimension of Daoism with its plethora of exercises, visualizations, ecstatic excursions, inner alchemy, and other meditations. Their practice can lead to enhanced vigor and longevity, but these are considered secondary when compared to their primary goal, the attainment of enlightenment and spiritual immortality.

The Chinese health program, thus, is not limited to one set of methods or practices, nor does it stop at healing patients and improving their quality of life. Rather, it leads people to reach extended years and to attain transcendence through refining the body into a new, more potent spirit existence.

At first glance these different dimensions seem to function on three entirely different levels of life. But from the Chinese perspective, healing, longevity, and immortality are three stages along the same continuum of the human body. The body consists of the cosmic vital energy of *qi*, which is only one but comes in two major forms: a basic primordial or prenatal *qi* that connects people to the cosmos; and a secondary, earthly or postnatal *qi* that is replenished by breathing, food, and human interaction, and helps the body survive in everyday life. Both forms of *qi* are necessary and interact constantly with each other, so that primordial *qi* is lost as and when earthly *qi* is insufficient, and earthly *qi* becomes superfluous as and when primordial *qi* is complete — as is the case with the embryo in the womb. People, once born, start an interchange of the two dimensions of *qi* and soon begin to lose their primordial *qi* as they interact with the world through shallow breathing, improper nutrition, emotional outbursts, sensory overloads, and intellectual tensions.

Once people have lost a certain amount of primordial *qi* and thus the power of their original, true self, they get sick and encounter difficulties in life and an impairment of health that will gradually lead to decline and death. Healing, then, is the replenishing of *qi* with medical means such as acupuncture, massages, diets, and herbs, combined with an increased awareness of *qi*-patterns and conscious lifestyle choices. Having attained good health, some people may decide to increase their primordial *qi* to the level they had at birth or even above it. To do so, they follow the longevity techniques to control their *qi*-exchange with the environment and cultivate themselves. The practice ensures the realization of people's natural life expectancy and often leads to increased old age and vigor.

Spiritual immortality, the goal of Daoism, raises the practices to a yet higher level. To attain it, people have to transform all their *qi* into primordial *qi* and proceed to refine it to subtler levels. This finer *qi* will eventually turn into pure spirit, with which practitioners increasingly identify to become transcendent spirit-people. The path that leads there involves intensive meditation and trance training as well as more radical forms of diet and other longevity practices. Immortality implies the overcoming of the natural tendencies of the body and its transformation into a different kind of *qi*-constellation. The result is a bypassing of death, so that the end of the body has no impact on the continuation of the spirit-person. In addition, practitioners attain supersensory powers and eventually gain residence in wondrous otherworldly paradises.

The very same kinds of practices may be used on all three levels, albeit in different ways and with caution. Certain practices that are useful in healing may be superfluous in the attainment of longevity, while some applicable for immortality may even be harmful when healing is the main focus. Take breathing as an example. When healing or extending life, natural deep breathing is emphasized, with the diaphragm expanding on the inhalation. When moving on to immortality, however, reversed breathing is advised, which means that the diaphragm contracts on the in-breath. Undertaking this kind of reversed breathing too early or at the wrong stage in one's practice can cause complications, from dizziness to disorientation or worse.

The same holds true in the case of sexual practices. In healing, sexual activity with a partner is encouraged in moderation, with both partners reaching regular climaxes. In longevity practice, sexual activity may still be performed with a partner, but ejaculation as a loss of *qi* is avoided and sexual stimulation is used to increase the positive flow of *qi* in the body. In immortality, finally, sexual practices are undertaken internally and without a partner. They serve the creation of an immortal embryo through the refinement of sexual energy into primordial *qi* and cosmic spirit. Going beyond nature, immortality practitioners are not interested in creating harmony and balance, but strive to overcome the natural tendencies of the body-mind and actively lessen or even relinquish earthly existence in favor of cosmic and heavenly states.

Encompassing this immense complexity and breadth, the Chinese vision of healing provides a clear set of answers to the urgent needs of modern Western patients. Unlike Western medicine, which has "scored its greatest successes when dealing not so much with human beings as with microorganisms at the lower end of the scale—namely, viruses and bacteria" (Porkert, *Chinese Medicine*, 55), Chinese medicine sees the larger picture of the human being in a cosmic and social context. It understands the essential unity and close correlation between body and mind, where Western doctors often still try to heal without taking emotions and thoughts into consideration. It deals with complex entities—the entire body, the person as a member of family and community—rather than with parts, such as livers, kidneys, or hearts. It is integrative, seeing the way different aspects work together, rather than reductionistic, trying to pinpoint the one single part that causes the disease or discomfort.

As a result, Eastern practitioners are general physicians. You will not typically find a "cardiac acupuncturist" or an herbalist specializing only in ailments of the liver, although in China today some practitioners have begun to specialize along the lines of Western biomedicine. Eastern doctors see every patient as a living whole and try to understand the exhibited symptoms in a synchronistic fashion. Without giving up the notion of the cause of a disease, they see this cause not in the defect of one part or the other, but find it in the pattern of interaction among the parts. Even these, however, they do not view as mere parts, like the mechanistic understanding of the body that tends to push and prod and ends up replacing faulty sections with artificially created or "harvested" ones. Instead, they understand each part of the body to be in constant exchange with all others and with everything else in society and the greater universe. All is in a state of dynamic flow, in an ongoing process.

Diagnosis accordingly is reached not so much with the help of machines but through human interaction and the observation of the patient as a whole and the appearance of his or her body in various critical areas, such as the tongue and the pulse. The subjective feelings of the patient are taken seriously into consideration — how often have you been told by a Western doctor that there is nothing wrong with you when you were clearly feeling out of sorts? What the doctor meant was that there was nothing *measurable* wrong with you, nothing he could detect on his numerical assays. The East Asian physician in contrast will place highest importance on your subjective feelings, measuring success less by the degree to which certain numbers on tests have "normalized" but by the amount of joy you are now able to experience. Quantity, without being totally disregarded, is placed secondary to quality; objective measuring gives way to subjective assessment.

Thus, the same symptom reported by two different people may lead to completely different diagnoses, since the patients' dynamic qi-flow is so different. Treatment, moreover, is not limited to the elimination of symptoms, which may result in a tendency to overtreat and has the danger of creating new ailments or side-effects, but aims at the overall increase in bodily vigor and enjoyment of life.

One problem, of course, with this emphasis on subjectivity and the personal flow of qi is that it is much harder to have controlled experiments on the efficacy of treatments or even double-blind studies. The moment anyone is placed in a laboratory environment, his natural tendencies are altered, and results from studies under artificial conditions cannot tell much about the techniques employed. To observe people in their natural, social environment, on the other hand, might yield results, but in our culture this tends to be more the prerogative of sociologists and psychologists than medical professionals. Still, it may also be worth doing, since understanding Chinese medicine properly and bringing it into the American and European mainstream will increase the awareness of lifestyle issues and enhance emphasis on prevention.

A greater attention to Chinese healing in the West may encourage doctors and patients to include emotional, psychological, and spiritual factors into the medical equation and create treatments that do not change symptoms but aim to restructure the underlying patterns. Instead of seeing illness as an alien force attacking an isolated entity such as a specific organ, people may come to understand it as a part of their reality that fulfills a certain function in their lives. Similarly, rather than considering pain as evil and suppress it with painkillers, they may see it as a signal of imbalance and the body's way of telling them that they need to make some changes to reconnect with themselves on a truer level.

Success can then be measured by the degree the patient is becoming responsible and balanced in his or her life and human interaction, finding not only health but happiness and good fortune. People may come to require more of themselves and their physicians in terms of well-being, no longer remaining content with getting through the day in the absence of symptoms. They may be empowered to understand their condition in holistic and dynamic terms, as part of a life-long process of learning and the unfolding of inherent potentials. Taking the initiative to find health, they may be motivated to make lasting changes in lifestyle and diet and commit to an exercise regimen that is appropriate for them and a joy to follow. Instead of tinkering with parts, they may work on themselves as a whole and aim at recovering their inherent perfection as part of heaven and earth, thus reaching out for the complete fullness of life.

Further Readings

Abramson, John. 2004. *Overdo$ed America: The Broken Promise of American Medicine*. New York: HarperCollins.

Eisenberg, David, and Thomas Lee Wright. 1985. *Encounters with Qi: Exploring Chinese Medicine*. New York: W. W. Norton & Co.

Larre, Claude, and Elisabeth Rochat de la Vallee. 1995. *Rooted in Spirit: The Heart of Chinese Medicine*. Translated by Sarah Stang. New York: Station Hill Press.

Porkert, Manfred, Mark Howson, and Christian Ullmann. 1988. *Chinese Medicine: As a Scientific System, Its History, Philosophy and Practice, and How it Fits With the Medicine of the West*. New York: Morrow.

Straten, N. H. van. 1983. *Concepts of Health, Disease and Vitality in Traditional Chinese Society*. Wiesbaden: Franz Steiner.

Chapter 1
Dao and Qi

The fundamental concept underlying Chinese healing is Dao, literally "the way." The term indicates the way things develop naturally, the way nature moves along and living beings grow and decline. The concept of Dao is not limited to Daoism, although the latter takes its name from it. Rather, it is part of the general Chinese understanding of the world, which appears in all different philosophical schools—albeit in slightly varying interpretations. This is why A.C. Graham calls his book on early Chinese philosophy *Disputers of the Dao*. Dao in this general sense is the one power underlying all. It makes things what they are and causes the world to come into being and decay. It is the fundamental ground of all: the motivation of evolution and the source of universal being.

The *Book of the Dao and Its Virtue* (*Daode jing*) says, "The Dao that can be told is not the eternal Dao" (ch. 1). Still, it is possible to create a working definition. Benjamin Schwartz, in his *The World of Thought in Ancient China*, describes the Dao as "organic order," organic in the sense that it is not willful, not a conscious, active creator or personal entity but an organic process that just moves along. But beyond this, Dao is also order—clearly manifest in the rhythmic changes and patterned processes of the natural world. As such it is predictable in its developments and can be discerned and described. Its patterns are what the Chinese call "self-so" or "nature" (*ziran*), the spontaneous and observable way things are naturally. Yet, while Dao is nature, it is also more than nature—its deepest essence, the inner quality that makes things what they are. It is governed by laws of nature, yet it is also these laws itself.

In other words, it is possible to explain the nature of the Dao in terms of a twofold structure. The "Dao that can be told" and the "eternal Dao." One is the mysterious, ineffable Dao at the center of the cosmos; the other is the Dao at the periphery, visible and tangible in the natural cycles of the known world. About the eternal Dao, the *Book of the Dao and Its Virtue* says:

> Look at it and do not see it: we call it invisible.
> Listen to it and do not hear it: we call it inaudible.
> Touch it and do not feel it: we call it subtle. . . .

Infinite and boundless, it cannot be named;
It belongs to where there are no beings.
It may be called the shape of no-shape,
It may be called the form of no-form.
Call it vague and obscure.
Meet it, yet you cannot see its head,
Follow it, yet you cannot see its back.
(ch. 14)

This Dao, although the ground and inherent power of the human being, is
entirely beyond ordinary perception.
Vague and obscure, it is beyond all
knowing and analysis; we cannot grasp
it however hard we try. The human
body, senses, and intellect are not
equipped to deal with it. The only way
a person can ever get in touch with it is
by forgetting and transcending ordinary
human faculties, by becoming subtler
and finer and more potent, more like
the Dao itself.

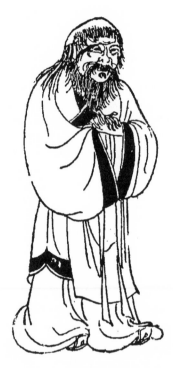

Fig. 1. Laozi, the alleged author of
the *Daode jing*.

The Dao at the periphery, on the other hand, is characterized as the give
and take of various pairs of complementary opposites, as the natural ebb
and flow of things as they rise and fall, come and go, grow and decline,
emerge and die. The *Book of the Dao and Its Virtue* says:

> To contract, there must first be expansion.
> To weaken, there must first be strengthening.
> To destroy, there must first be promotion.
> To grasp, there must first be giving.
> This is called the subtle pattern. (ch. 36)

Things develop in alternating movements as long as they live. It is the
nature of life to be in constant motion. Things always move in one direction or the other: up or down, toward lightness or heaviness, brightness
or darkness. Nature is a continuous flow of becoming, whether latent or
manifest, described as the alternation of complementary characteristics

and directions that cannot exist without each other. This becoming can be rhythmic and circular, or it can move back toward the source of life in the ineffable Dao, which at the same time is a forward movement toward a new level of cosmic oneness.

Within this dual-layered universe of the Dao, ineffable at the center and manifest in natural rhythms at the periphery, the second most essential concept of Chinese health and long life is *qi*. *Qi* is the concrete aspect of the Dao, the material energy of the universe, the basic stuff of nature. In ancient sources it is associated with mist, fog, and moving clouds. The character for *qi* as it appears in the oracle bones of the Shang dynasty (1766-1122 B.C.E.), consists of two parts: an image of someone eating and grain in a pot. Combined, these parts signal *qi*, the quality which nourishes, warms, transforms, and rises. *Qi*, therefore, is contained in the foods we eat and the air we breathe. But more subtly it is also the life force in the human body and as such is the basis of all physical vitality.

By extension, *qi* also denotes anything perceptible but intangible: atmosphere, smoke, aroma, vapor, a sense of intuition, foreboding, or even ghosts. There is only one *qi*, just as there is only one Dao. But it, too, appears on different levels of subtlety and in different modes. At the center, there is primordial *qi*, prenatal *qi*, or true, perfect *qi*; at the periphery, there is postnatal *qi* or earthly *qi*—like the measurable Dao it is in constant motion and divided according to categories such as temperature, density, speed of flow, and impact on human life.

Qi is the basic material of all that exists. It animates life and furnishes functional power of events. *Qi* is the root of the human body; its quality and movement determine human health. *Qi* can be discussed in terms of quantity, since having more means stronger metabolic function. This, however, does not mean that health is a byproduct of storing large quantities of *qi*. Rather, there is a normal or healthy amount of *qi* in every person, and health manifests in its balance and harmony, its moderation and smoothness of flow. This flow is envisioned in the texts as a complex system of waterways with the "Ocean of *Qi*" in the abdomen; rivers of *qi* flowing through the upper torso, arms, and legs; springs of *qi* reaching to the wrists and ankles; and wells of *qi* found in the fingers and toes. Even a small spot in this complex system can thus influence the whole, so that overall balance and smoothness are the general goal.

Human life is the accumulation of *qi*; death is its dispersal. After receiving a core potential of primordial *qi* at birth, people throughout life need to sustain it. They do so by drawing postnatal *qi* into the body from air and food, as well as from other people through sexual, emotional, and social interaction. But they also lose *qi* through breathing bad air, over-burdening their bodies with food and drink, and getting involved in negative emotions and excessive sexual or social interactions.

It is thus best to breathe deeply and to eat moderately in accordance with the seasons, to move smoothly, exercise without exertion, and match activities to the body's needs. This is how one keeps balance and creates health. As the *Spring and Autumn Annals of Master Lü* (*Lüshi chunqiu*), a text from about 260 B.C.E., has it:

> One wants the skin to be tight, the blood vessels to allow un-impeded motion; the sinews to be firm and the bones hard; the heart, mind, and will to be concordant; and the vital energies to flow. When this is happening, agents of disorder [sickness] have nowhere to abide and pathology has nowhere to be produced. The abiding of agents of sickness is the origin of pathology, which is blocking the flow of *qi*. (ch. 4)

Health is not just the absence of symptoms and ailments. It is the presence of a strong vital energy and of a smooth, harmonious, and active flow of *qi*. This is known as the state of *zhengqi* or "proper *qi*," also translated as "upright *qi*." The ideal is to have *qi* flow freely, thereby creating harmony in the body and a balanced state of being in the person. This personal health is further matched by health in nature, defined as regular weather patterns and the absence of disasters. It is also present as health in society in the peaceful coexistence among families, clans, villages, and states. This harmony on all levels, the cosmic presence of a steady and pleasant flow of *qi*, is what the Chinese call the state of Great Peace (*taiping*), a state venerated by Confucians and Daoists alike.

The opposite of health is *xieqi* or "wayward *qi*," also called "deviant *qi*," "pathogenic *qi*," "heteropathic *qi*," or "evil *qi*." All these expressions are used in Western textbooks to translate the same Chinese term. The variety reflects the different views of the translators and shifts the meaning of the term and thereby the understanding of what goes on in the body. Typically, medical or Latin-based words like "heteropathic" tend to be more technical and overshadow the moral implications of the original term, while words like "evil" or "deviant" have moral and social rather than medical implications.

Xieqi or "wayward *qi*" is *qi* that has lost the harmonious pattern of flow and no longer supports the dynamic forces of change. Whereas *zhengqi* moves in a steady, harmonious rhythm and effects daily renewal, helping health and long life, *xieqi*, disorderly and dysfunctional, creates change that violates the normal order. When it becomes dominant, the *qi*-flow can turn upon itself and deplete the body's resources. The patient no longer operates as part of a universal system and is not in tune with the basic life force around him or her. *Xieqi* appears when *qi* begins to move either too fast or too slow, is excessive or depleted, or creates rushes or obstructions. It disturbs the regular flow and causes ailments.

Qi can become excessive through outside influences such as too much heat or cold or through inside patterns such as too much emotion or stimulation. Excessive *qi* can be moving too fast or be very sluggish, as in the case of excessive dampness. Whatever the case, from a universal perspective there is no extra or new *qi* created, but localized disharmonies have arisen because existing *qi* has become excessive and thus harmful. Still, even describing it in this way we are thinking in terms of *qi* as an energetic substance, which it really is not. A better way to speak of it would be to say that the process itself of turning hot or angry is *qi*, that the way things move and change is what constitutes our being *qi*.

Similarly, *qi* can be in depletion. This may mean that there is a tense flow of *qi* due to nervousness or anxiety, or that the volume and density of *qi* have decreased, which is the case in serious prolonged illness. However, more commonly it means that the *qi* activity level is lower, that its flow is not quite up to standard, that there is a lower than normal concentration of *qi* in one or the other body part. In the same vein, perfection of *qi* means the optimal functioning of energy in the body, while control of *qi* means the power to guide the energetic process to one or the other part.

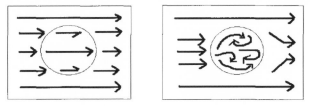

Fig. 2. The proper and wayward flow of *qi*.

To conceptualize *qi* in the body, imagine a fluid-filled sack under water. The sack has a semi-permeable membrane: it can absorb the external fluid and excrete fluid out. The water surrounding the sack has waves that also influence its inner fluids. Viewed from a bird's-eye perspective as an integrated system, every wave and eddy in both sack and water are "upright" or "correct," because that is just how things are. However, within the smaller system of the sack there is a microcosm of flow which can be out of balance. This imbalance can come from exposure to certain aspects of the greater flow which causes the internal flow to become overly committed to one specific pattern. Or it could be that the fluid in the sack has too much or too little internal substance, and is thus unable to keep up with external patterns. Whichever it is, the uncooperative flow within the smaller sack is *xieqi* or "wayward *qi*." From a universal perspective, any flow is just flow. From the perspective of the individual body, some flow may be wayward because correctness (health) is the desired state.

> **Exercise:** Find your own metaphors for the functioning of *qi*. What image works for you? How can you get a personal sense of this force and its activity?

For the Chinese system, this means that healing is the correction of *qi*-flow from a deviant or wayward pattern back to a harmonious or correct flow, matching the rhythm of the Dao on the periphery, creating health and well-being in the person, and aiding him or her in familial and professional interactions. Longevity is the enhancement and strengthening of the proper flow of *qi*, allowing people to fully go along with all the movements of the manifest Dao in order to enjoy health, retain vigor, and live long and successful lives. Immortality, finally, is the move toward the Dao at the center, the transformation of a proper, healthy, and harmonious *qi* into the subtler levels of cosmic energy, into a mysterious and ineffable state of being that goes far beyond the natural world.

To understand *qi* properly, we need to realize that it functions in subtle forms and activities and that, therefore, it should not be described in terms of substance or as a limited "energy." Rather, the way *qi* works should be expressed in terms of relationships and correspondences, in terms of what it does and how it impacts cosmos and self. *Qi* is process. The way to describe health and sickness accordingly is by speaking not about an existing quality but about the way things function.

In this respect Chinese medical worldview is not unlike that of modern physics. Here chaos theory describes the way things work in terms of a well-functioning natural control system marked by a fair degree of unpredictability; a constant chance for new possibilities and new discoveries; an unceasing process of movement, change, and transformation. This transformation, moreover, is described in terms of quantum fields which, unlike gravity or magnetism, carry neither matter nor energy.

Quantum physics states that the subatomic world is in no way like the world we inhabit. Energy is not continuous, but instead comes in small units: quanta, the energy that electrons absorb or emit when changing energy levels; and gluons, the forces that hold atoms together. The most basic subatomic particles behave like both particles and waves, and many of these particles form pairs like yin and yang, where one cannot exist without the other. The movement, moreover, of these particles is inherently random. It is impossible to know both the exact momentum and location of a particle at the same time — in fact, there is an inverse relationship in that the more information one has about the former, the less is known about the latter, and vice versa (see http://phys.educ. ksu.edu).

Quantum physics has shown that matter is made up of vibrating energy and fields which change their state very rapidly — trillions of times in one second. Atoms are largely empty and consist of a tiny nucleus that is ten thousand times smaller than the rest of the particle — 99,999 parts being emptiness. Body and mind consist of the same vibrating atoms that are constantly oscillating, arising and dissolving: all empty, no solidity, no firmness. As a result, reality has to be understood less as the combination of solid entities than as an interlocking web of fields that each pulsate at their own rate. These interlocking fields of vibration — described in China as patterns of qi-flow — can come into harmony with each other and mutually support and increase their amplitude. But they can also interfere with each other and create disturbance. Since all fields are ultimately interlocked, even a small disturbance in any one of them carries into all the others. This holds true not only for the body, but also integrates the mind into a vibrational body-mind totality. Just as bodily transformations are of unlimited possibilities, so the mind is ultimately non-local; it can be anywhere and exchange information with anything else instantaneously (see www.newscientist.com/hottopics/quantum).

The body-mind continuum is also at the root of the understanding of qi in Chinese cosmology, which explains it in terms of vibration and sound and which states that all existing things consist of qi-flow and have form or shape which inevitably vibrates at a certain frequency, creating a certain wave pattern and a specific sound. As a result, the entire universe is humming along in the joining of many different qi-sounds. The *Book of Master Zhuang* (*Zhuangzi*; ca. 250 B.C.E.) accordingly talks about the "piping of humanity," the sounds people make when they speak and interact; the "piping of earth," the sounds of nature in all the different places on the planet; and the "piping of heaven" the creation of the universe in its diversity through the Dao. The description of the "piping of earth" is most vivid and also applies to the other forms. The text says:

> They roar like waves, whistle like arrows, screech, gasp, cry, wail, moan, howl. Those in the lead cry out *yeee*; those behind cry out *yuuu*. In a gentle breeze, they answer faintly; but in a full gale, the chorus is gigantic. And when the fierce wind has passed on, then all the hollows are empty again. Have you never seen the tossing and trembling that goes on? (ch. 2)

The formation of pathology follows the same paradigm of the cosmic creation of sounds and vibrations through the movement of *qi*. "Wind is the cause of the hundred diseases," the *Yellow Emperor's Inner Classic* (*Huangdi neijing*) says. "It enters the body and exhausts human *qi*," mingling with "the eight winds in heaven and the five winds in the arteries of the body."

A similar view of the universe as a conglomeration of vibrating, closely interconnected entities is also found in modern physics. As Itzhak Bentov describes it in his *Stalking the Wild Pendulum*, all is constantly surrounded by sound. Sound can appear as random acoustic disturbances, such as voices, body, hand, or air movements, or again in rhythmic patterns as a note, a single acoustic frequency (*Pendulum*, 23). An experiment known both to the ancient Chinese and modern physicists is the harmony created among two string instruments. If you pluck the string of one lute, the matching string on a lute sitting next to it will begin to vibrate. Similarly, if you apply the violin bow to sheet metal with sand, you get a distinctive pattern of standing waves or nodal points that form both active and quiescent areas. These show the pattern of *qi* in the universe, the alteration between ups and downs, activity and rest.

Exercise: Go to http://phys.educ.ksu.edu/vqm/html/wpe.html and examine the experiment on the behavior of wave patterns. How can their nature be relevant to our world? How would its adoption into your thinking change your vision of self and life?

Smooth *qi*-flow is thus essentially entrainment or vibrational harmony among different objects or parts of the same entity. Various modes are possible. Superimpose two sounds of identical wave pattern: hill matches hill, valley matches valley, and the amplitude of the original wave pattern is doubled. This is called constructive interference or the "productive" pattern of qi-interaction. Superimpose two sounds of opposite wave pattern: the exact opposite happens, they cancel each other out and the wave vanishes into a straight line. This is disruptive interference, the creation of disharmony and a "destructive" form of qi- interaction.

In the case of varying wavelengths, moreover, some phases match each other while others do not. This results in a curve that goes up and down, is far apart at one point, then meets again and parts again. A rhythmic pattern of interaction emerges, typical for the natural and human world. This, in turn, matches not only the classical view of the movements of Dao and qi in the Chinese universe, but also modern physics. As described by David Bohm in *Quantum Theory*, living organisms are intrinsically dynamic. Their visible forms are nothing but apparently stable manifestations of underlying processes that change continuously in rhythmic patterns—fluctuations, oscillations, vibrations, waves.

The ideal of harmonious qi-flow and entrained vibrations, then, is a completely resonant system. The waves of one entity impinge on another so that it moves in the same frequency. This, in essence, is the definition of health in Chinese culture. The qi-vibrations of each body part resonate smoothly with all others. We as people resonate harmoniously with the people and things around us; society and nature resonate perfectly with each other. The ideal of Great Peace, the total harmony of Dao, is reached when all beings and things hum on the same wavelength and frequency, in a state of optimum transfer and total resonance.

In terms of medicine, this means that the body is a conglomeration of various vibratory fields. Never can there be just one single cause for a given symptom, but the interconnection of the whole needs to be examined. Nor can the body be viewed in isolation, but should be seen in relation to the many fields outside: planets, earth, society, family, and so on. Disease and disorder may be related to the out-of-tune behavior of one or the other section in the flow of vibration, but they affect the whole and can be approached from many different angles. Corrections come accordingly in various forms and should have an effect on the entirety of the system, applying a strong harmonizing rhythm to any given part of the vibration pattern. Eventually the flow moves back into its harmonious rhythm and health is recovered.

To sum up, the body, society, nature, and the planetary fields can be imagined as a huge bowl of fairly rigid jelly with raisins in it (Bentov,

Pendulum, 29). Vibrate one part of it, and the rest also vibrates. One section cannot move without the other, and even the slightest touch to one single raisin will immediately transmit movements to all the others and the body of the jelly—a concept the Chinese describe as "impulse and response" (*ganying*). The same also holds true for human bodies. We all have electrical charges in and around us, which are measurable and can be felt. The Chinese see these charges as the body's *qi*-field which not only interacts with the organs and parts on its inside but also with the electric field of things around it and the planet at large—a field that is weaker but still present. Through systematic *qi*-enhancement practices, people can achieve a fully tuned system that not only is very healthy but may attain long life and even immortality.

Further Readings

Bentov, Itchak. 1977. *Stalking the Wild Pendulum: On the Mechanics of Consciousness*. New York: E. P. Dutton.

Bohm, David. 1951. *Quantum Theory*. New York: Prentice-Hall.

Capra, Fritjof. 1975. *The Tao of Physics: An Exploration of the Parallels Between Modern Physics and Eastern Mysticism*. Boulder: Shambhala.

Fung Yu-lan. 1952. *A History of Chinese Philosophy*. Translated by Derk Bodde. 2 vols. Princeton: Princeton University Press.

Gerber, Richard. 1988. *Vibrational Medicine: New Choices for Healing Ourselves*. Santa Fe: Bear and Company.

Graham, A. C. 1989. *Disputers of the Tao: Philosophical Argument in Ancient China*. La Salle, Ill.: Open Court Publishing Company.

Gribbin, John. 1984. *In Search of Schrödinger's Cat*. Toronto: Bantam Books.

Puett, Michael. 2002. *To Become a God: Cosmology, Sacrifice, and Self-Divinization in Early China*. Cambridge, Mass.: Harvard University Press.

Schwartz, Benjamin. 1985. *The World of Thought in Ancient China*. Cambridge, Mass.: Harvard University Press.

Slingerland, Edward. 2003. *Effortless Action: Wu-wei as Conceptual Metaphor and Spiritual Ideal in Early China*. New York: Oxford University Press.

Zukav, Gary. 1979. *The Dancing Wuli Masters: An Overview of the New Physics*. New York: Bantam.

Chapter 2
Yin-Yang and the Five Phases

To achieve physical wellness and spiritual perfection, one must first understand how the Dao works at the periphery, how *qi* flows in its most obvious patterns. The way the Chinese have described this reality is in terms of "phase energetics," i.e., as movements of energy and flowing forces classified into specific types and phases. Two models stand out—the interchange of the two forces of yin and yang and the various interaction cycles of the five phases.

Yin and yang are at the root of traditional Asian cosmology. "One yin, one yang, that is the Dao," says the *Book of Changes* (*Yijing*), the ancient divination manual of the Zhou dynasty (1122-221 B.C.E.) that still serves to tell fortunes today. Yin and yang are commonly presented in the well-known circle with two black and white curved halves, plus a white dot in the black section and a black dot in the white section. The image shows the balance and yet interlocking nature of yin and yang, the fluidity of their interchange.

The amount of white or black on each side of the diagram starts narrow and becomes wider, then ends in a narrow line. Where the white part is largest, the black begins to emerge. This shows how the two change into each other, how yang emerges at the highest point of yin, and vice versa. The symbol emphasizes the need for being inclusive and whole, to strive for balance yet be ready to change. Yin and yang form the bipolar base of a complex system of correspondences, a numerical way to explain the world. They provide the organizing concepts for the ancient proto-sciences, such as astronomy, music, divination, and medicine (see www.chinese medicinesampler.com).

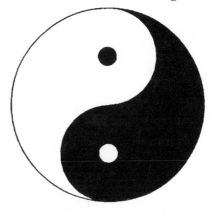

Fig. 3. The classic symbol of yin and yang.

Their underlying structure is a form of correlative thinking, which is not unique to China but can also be found in other traditional cultures, such as ancient Greece, and in the West is still used in occultism and magic. It represents a basic pattern of the human mind, forms the foundation of more elaborate forms of logic, and is clearly present in the way we acquire language. For example, to build the plural of *shoe*, we add the letter "s" to get *shoes*. The same applies to cat/cats, stone/stones, road/roads. But then we learn that this correlative pattern when applied to the word *foot* is wrong and instead of *foots* we use another pattern and go from *foot* to *feet*, then apply the same to get goose/geese, and so on. In all cases, the organization of language is based on a simple pattern that is correlated and repeated in different concrete cases (Graham, *Yin-Yang*).

The correlative system of understanding also comes into play in a more general understanding of reality. For example, the working of the human body may be applied to politics, so that the mind in relation to the body is understood as similar to the ruler's relation to his subjects. A more mechanical vision of the body may see the relation of mind to body as that of governor engine to other engines. In all these cases, similarities and differences between patterns are recognized and reality is understood in terms of the interaction of different aspects that impact on each other. In a next step, the correlation pattern itself creates a specific vision of reality—as correlated and interactive—and thus new realities are formed on the basis of further association. These patterns tend to work particularly within a given culture and among people who share a common paradigm. Over time, this paradigm shifts, allowing for new correlations and models to take over.

Chinese cosmology is based on correlative thinking. It emphasizes the dynamic interaction among fields and integrated patterns. Based on a different understanding of the structure of the world than Western linear analysis that focuses on logic and the law of cause and effect, correlative thinking is more ancient and more fundamental than science. This, however, does not mean that it does not allow a high level of sophistication. Correspondences can be very elaborate, support advanced technology, and retain some causal forms of explanation. Beyond all this, though, they have the advantage of providing an integrated explanation for the entire cosmos and preventing reductionist and particularistic thinking.

Yang and yin originated from geographical observation, indicating the sunny and shady sides of a hill. From there they acquired a series of associations: bright and dark, light and heavy, strong and weak, above and below, heaven and earth, ruler and minister, male and female, and so on.

In concrete application, moreover, they indicate different kinds of action:

yang	active	birth	impulse	move	change	expansion
yin	structive	completion	response	rest	nurture	contraction

These characteristics were in turn associated with items in daily life:

yang	heaven	spring	summer	day	big states	ruler	man
yin	earth	fall	winter	night	small states	minister	woman

Father	life	unfolding	noble	marriage	soldiers	speech	give
mother	death	stagnation	common	funeral	laborers	silence	receive

It may at first glance seem that yang is "better" than yin. In the Chinese view, however, neither is better, stronger, brighter, or more preferable, and the two forces do not represent good and evil. On the contrary, the yin aspect of things is just as important as the yang, because you cannot have one without other. They are not opposites but complementary phases of *qi*-flow, one bringing forth the other in close mutual interdependence (see http://asiarecipe.com/yinyang.html).

Yin-yang thinking comes with its own kind of logic. For example, why do fire and sun radiate outside, while water and moon seem to absorb inward? Because to illuminate is to expel *qi*, to retreat to the dark is to contain it. Or again, why are animals and birds yang, invertebrates and fish yin? Because the former run and fly, the latter hibernate and hide. Why, when disturbed, do birds fly up but fish dive down? Because fire goes up and water goes down. There is, thus, a distinct logic in this thinking of phase energetics that sees things moving and developing in particular ways.

> **Exercise:** List as many correlations of yin and yang as you can. Think of everything you do in daily life in terms of yin and yang: resting and rising, brushing and spitting, chewing and swallowing, moving and resting.

The yin-yang system provides a good working basis for understanding the patterns of the Dao on the periphery and seeing the concrete manifestations of *qi*-flow in the course of ordinary life. It is yet made more complex and more sophisticated by a subdivision into five phases: minor yang—major yang—yin/yang—minor yin—major yin.

In other words, the rhythmic pattern of rise and decline in the structure of energetic exchange is finely tuned. To use the rise and dips of hills and valleys as a metaphor, as you climb the hill, coming out of the valley, the sun will hit you just a little bit, there is slight warmth and light, or yang in its minor phase. As you go up the hill, the sun will get brighter, the views will be broader, the overall feeling more expansive, and you come to the major phase of yang. After reaching the top, as you begin descend, there is a balance between yin and yang, neither one nor the other. Then, as you go down further, the light gets less, views are more restricted, you feel a decline—you are in the phase of minor yin. As you eventually reach the bottom of the valley, with its greater darkness, coolness, and shadiness, your path evens out for a while and you are in the state of major yin. From here, sooner or later, as you walk along, the terrain will rise again and the cycle repeats. It is in constant motion, and one part necessarily follows from the other.

This phase system of five minor and major stages of yin and yang is then linked with five organic substances that symbolize the different stages in the process:

minor yang	major yang	yin-yang	minor yin	major yin
wood	fire	earth	metal	water

These are known as the "five phases" (*wuxing*). They are often also referred to as the "five elements," because they have a superficial similarity with the Greek or Indian elements—water, fire, earth, and air. However, properly speaking the appellation "element" is incorrect, since unlike in India and Greece where they refer to solid substances and firm, unchanging building blocks of the world, in China they indicate phase energetics and dynamic processes in a constant state of transformation.

Historically, the five phases underwent several stages of development. They are first documented in the *Book of History* (*Shujing*), an ancient record dating from about 800 B.C.E. Here they appear as the "five materials" and are concrete substances, resources used for human livelihood. They are, at this stage, not *qi* at all—*qi* is found in sunshine, shade, moonlight, vapors, and other atmospheric conditions—but substances that people actually use. As such, they should be treated with care and used with moderation and wisdom. They are offered to the gods on the altars of soil and grain, and they have to be guarded by rulers to ensure their continued productivity without excess or deficiency.

In their natural rhythm, the five materials produce each other continuously in a harmonious cycle. Thus, water comes about through rainfall. It makes things grow, so that there is lush vegetation and wood arises. Wood dries and becomes fuel for fire, which burns and creates ashes. Ashes become earth, and earth over long periods of consolidation grows metals in its depths. Metals in the depths of mountains, moreover, attract clouds and stimulate rainfall, thus closing the cycle.

At the same time, however, the five materials also serve as a system of mutual control or checks and balances, keeping things in their proper order. Thus, water can extinguish fire, fire can melt metal, metal can cut wood, wood can contain earth, earth can dam water, and water can again extinguish fire. Here the inherently dynamic nature of the five materials is not used to increase productivity, but to set boundaries and limit potential excesses. In all cases, the early vision emphasizes that although the five materials are substances for human use, they are not merely innate objects but contain dynamic powers that can be turned both to production or control.

In another chapter of the *Book of History* entitled "The Great Plan," the five materials are treated in a slightly more abstract manner and associated more with qualities, processes, and psychological factors. Wood is linked with the qualities of bending and straightness, fire with flaming and rising, earth with planting and harvesting, metal with being formable and sharp, and water with wetting and sinking. These, in turn, are associated with five activities and five attitudes:

wood	fire	earth	metal	water
hearing	seeing	demeanor	thinking	speech
perceptive	clear	respectful	understanding	appropriate

This early association of the five materials with qualities and human psychology laid an important foundation for later developments. It represents the beginning of the mature system as it became central in Chinese culture. Expanding this early model of the five materials, the cosmologist Zou Yan (4th c. B.C.E.) created the concept of the "five powers" or "five virtues" by focusing on the potency inherent in the materials, such as wood's power to grow and be lush and fire's power to flame and rise. He then correlated these abstract powers with the political dynamics of succeeding dynasties, linking his own Zhou dynasty with fire, and predicted that it would be overcome by a newly arising ruler who would conquer it through the symbolic power of water—following the controlling cycle of the five materials.

This system was picked up by later cosmologists who created a great, encompassing scheme of dynastic succession. It also led to extensive predictions and uprisings, during which revolutionaries dressed in colors associated with the rising phase and claimed that their time to rule had come. In addition, ruling dynasties subscribed to their associated "power" by dressing officials in its colors, using the multiples of its numbers as measuring systems, and generally aligning with it.

Beyond the political sphere, the five powers of Zou Yan became the foundation of the five phases proper, a complex, integrated cosmological system that fully developed in the early Han dynasty around 200 B.C.E. At this time the five energetic phases were associated not only with colors, but also with directions, seasons, musical tones, and with various functions in the human body, such as yin organs, yang organs, senses, emotions, and flavors. The basic chart, which has been at the root of Chinese cosmology ever since and also forms the diagnostic and analytical foundation of the Chinese health system is as follows:

yin/yang	phase	direct.	color	season	organ1	organ2	emotion	sense
minor yang	wood	east	green	spring	liver	gall	anger	eyes
major yang	fire	south	red	summer	heart	sm. int.	exc. joy	tongue
yin-yang	earth	center	yellow		spleen	stomach	worry	lips
minor yin	metal	west	white	fall	lungs	lg. int.	sadness	nose
major yin	water	north	black	winter	kidneys	bladder	fear	ears

This set of correspondences served predominantly to identify relationships. In the official sphere it was used to explain why certain actions should be undertaken in certain seasons. For example, it became a general rule that because heaven and earth make the myriad creatures blossom in spring, one should in that season sleep and rise early, loosen the hair, relax the body, and allow all beings to live, abstaining from killing. Spring was a time of giving and not of taking, of reward and not of punishment. By following these injunctions, humanity was believed to act in proper alignment with the *qi* of spring and to secure health and harmony for both body and society. Any actions against the dominant *qi*-flow, on the other hand, would cause harm to the liver, the organ associated with wood and spring, and would create chills in the summer. They might also arouse aggression and anger, the corresponding emotions, and make for social upheaval and unhappiness.

Exercise: Given the above chart, how would injunctions for the other three seasons look like? Can you outline proper seasonal behavior for summer, fall, and winter?

In other words, the correspondence system provides a vision of the universe that is relational and dynamic, since it conceives of all social, physical, and psychological occurrences in terms of natural cycles and ongoing patterns. It places human beings in a world that is not, as in modern science, governed by invariable laws but subject to a pattern of interaction that can be either orderly or chaotic. It thereby both limits and empowers people. It limits them by placing them into a natural cycle which responds to what they do and puts on them the demand of total adaptation for success and fulfillment. Yet it also empowers them because it gives them an active role in the interaction with all things, the power to either support or disturb the natural and political order.

Adopting the relational scheme first developed in conjunction with the five materials, the five phases with all their cosmological complexity similarly follow a productive and a controlling cycle—also known as the generative, creative, or *sheng* cycle and the conquest, control, or *ke* cycle (www.kehper.net/topics/eastern/wuxing.html; www.lieske.com). The cycles are as follows:

Productive: wood – fire – earth – metal – water (1 2 3 4 5)

Controlling: wood – earth – water – fire – metal (1 3 5 2 4)

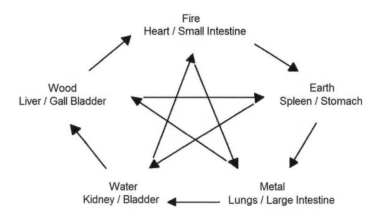

Fig. 4. The five phases in their various sequences.

The productive sequence shows the production of *qi*-flow through the various phases and their associated organs, emotions, and so on. Each phase provides for the next like a mother for her child. Not only applied to human behavior throughout the year and to the timing of political measures, it plays an important part in medical diagnostics. If one part in this chain is weak, the sequence shows how the weakness passes on to the next and explains why, for example, someone with symptoms typically associated with the lungs has in fact a weakness of the spleen. To treat the condition, one begins by stimulating and harmonizing the organ showing the symptoms, then gradually moves back toward the organ of origin.

The controlling sequence, also known as the conquest cycle, is similarly used in diagnosis. It is a representation of the catabolic ability of the body. It is necessary for the body not to overproduce. If a given phase fails to control the next, there may be stagnation, obstruction, or an excessive flow of *qi* in the uncontrolled phase. If one phase controls another too much, there will be a deficiency in the controlled phase.

In addition, although more rarely, diagnosis also operates with reversed sequences:

Reversed production: wood — water — metal — earth — fire (1 5 4 3 2)

Reversed control: wood — metal — fire — water — earth (1 4 2 5 3)

In the reversed production cycle, too much in one phase prevents the earlier one from doing its job, and the weakness moves backwards. In the reversed control sequence, there is a violation, so that if one phase is deficient, the one following conquers it and encroaches on it. This violates all the others in a backward movement.

For example, a patient presents with heart trouble. If the cause is immediately in the heart, it is probably fire-related and straightforward to diagnose. If it is not immediately in the heart, but the heart symptoms are secondary to problems in another area, it can be diagnosed either through the production or control sequences. According to the production sequence, wood produces fire, thus the liver is the mother organ of the heart. If the transmission follows this line, from mother to child, it is called a "deficiency pattern" and needs repletion or tonifying treatment. If the movement of *qi* goes the other way, in a backward motion from the child to the mother, in this case from earth to fire or spleen to heart, then it is called a "repletion pattern" and needs to be drained and depleted.

According to the controlling cycle, water conquers fire, and therefore the kidneys could be the ultimate cause of the heart trouble. This is known as a "controlling cycle disharmony." If the reverse motion is the case, however, and the lungs are pushing the control back toward the heart, we speak of an "insulting cycle disharmony." This is more difficult to treat. In each case, the specific cause and relationship among the various organs is found through detailed diagnosis which also includes the patient's preferences or excesses in terms of colors, tastes, emotions, climates, seasons, and so on. Then usually a combination of treatments to both symptom and cause organ is administered. The goal of establishing the various patterns is to set each organ into a relationship with all the others, providing a system with which to explain the manifestation of multiple, maybe even contradictory, indicators in a given diagnosis.

> **Exercise:** A patient comes in with a pattern of liver disharmony. Describe the possible five-phases patterns which could account for this problem.

Another level of application of the five phases system in health practice is the determination of constitutional and personality types, which is documented in ancient China in physiognomic texts, i.e., materials on fortune-telling with the help of body shapes and facial complexion. In the West, this system was especially developed in the French school of acupuncture, and described by Yves Requena. According to him, each phase corresponds to one constitution, including a particular body shape, which is vulnerable primarily in one specific organ and shows typical childhood symptoms, adult illnesses, and likes and dislikes.

For example, a person of the wood constitution has wide shoulders and good muscles, a greenish complexion, large eyes, wide eyebrows, and well-proportioned limbs. He or she has a natural weakness in the liver and gallbladder, tends toward allergies and nervousness as a child, and shows skin and digestive problems as an adult. A person of the fire constitution similarly has a slender body, reddish complexion, and long, slender hands. He or she has a leaning toward trouble in the heart or small intestine, is prone to psychological instability both as a child and as an adult, dreads the summer heat, but enjoys bitter flavors (see Requena, *Character and Health*).

Expanding this system, acupuncturist Jason Elias created a model where not only physical but also psychological personality patterns are matched with the five phases. According to him, the wood person is commanding and organized; the fire person is vibrant, loving, and full of enthusiasm; the earth person is centered, giving, and a born peacemaker; the metal person is straightforward, mystical, and artistic; and the water person is visionary, thoughtful, and philosophical. In each case, the dominant pattern can appear in excess or deficiency, leading to overly controlling, restless, or dependent forms of behavior. There are certain diets, supplements, exercises, and meditations for each type that will help restore balance (see Elias, *The Five Elements of Self-Healing*).

Yet a different take on this understanding of the five phases, which also includes the theories of British acupuncturist J. R. Worsley, is presented by acupuncturist Lonny Jarrett. He identifies certain attitudes in life and basic problems that people have to face in order to determine their key area of healing and fulfillment of destiny. As he says:

> In general, the foundation of all spiritual development is to first set the will on wanting freedom more than anything else. Once the will is set in this way, our choices in life are clarified. In this regard we should help the patient make a connection between what he complains about (his symptoms) and his dysfunctional beliefs, thoughts, and behaviors. In short, it is important to educate the patient regarding everything else he is choosing other than health. (*Clinical Practice*, 63)

For example, in classical Chinese cosmology, the phase water is associated with the kidneys and the bladder. Emotionally it is linked with fear, its main psychological agent is the will, and its key virtue is wisdom. According to Jarrett, people of this type respond to fear by overusing their wills, which depletes their resources and particularly their essence. This in turn leads to weakness in the bones and the nervous system, which encourages more fear. They vacillate between conformity—the need to go along with the demands of society and to work within the limitations of their physical ability and social position—and their ideal vision of themselves, moving between phases of extreme anxiety and recklessness, between overcoming and denying their fear.

Similarly, fire people with their heart-based constitution face a strong conflict between chaos (a loose heart) and control (a tight heart), the pursuit of pleasure and extreme measures to avoid sorrow. People dominated by wood face issues of belligerence versus timidity, situations where they can move forward aggressively versus times when they hardly dare to set foot out of their house, which leads to times of excessive planning and strong forward pushes versus periods of stagnation and a sense of frustration. People of dominantly metal constitution face a strong tension between grief for things past and longing for the future. They do not know when to let go and when to hang on, when to move ahead and when to stay put. Earth people, finally, tend to struggle with issues of service versus selfishness, personal needs versus being needed by others. In all cases, resolution of the conflict involves a strengthening of the appropriate virtue and a greater balance of forces.

These various personality types are a modern development of the ancient system of the five phases, based on clinical experience and a great deal of reading in the spiritual literature of ancient China. They go beyond the mere healing of symptoms and diseases to the identification of fundamental issues of destiny—things that people are meant to deal with in this life and that they need to resolve to realize themselves to the fullest. All other symptoms, using the various dynamic sequences of the five phases, in this system are seen as secondary to the ultimate issue and are treated one by one, to eventually open the path for people to find greater self-realization. It is not surprising, then, that Jarrett's treatments take years rather than months and involve major changes not only in dietary and bodily habits but in lifestyle and the overall direction of life.

Further Readings

Chan, Wing-tsit. 1963. *A Source Book in Chinese Philosophy*. Princeton: Princeton University Press.

Elias, Jason, and Katherine Ketcham. 1998. *The Five Elements of Self-Healing: Using Chinese Medicine for Maximum Immunity, Wellness, and Health*. New York: Harmony Books.

Fung Yu-lan. 1952. *A History of Chinese Philosophy*. Translated by Derk Bodde. 2 vols. Princeton, Princeton University Press.

Graham, A. C. 1986. *Yin-Yang and the Nature of Correlative Thinking*. Singapore: The Institute for East Asian Philosophies.

Hammer, Leo. 1990. *Dragon Rises, Red Bird Flies: Psychology and Chinese Medicine*. Barrytown, NY: Station Hill Press.

Jarrett, Lonny S. 2000. *Nourishing Destiny: The Inner Tradition of Chinese Medicine*. Stockbridge: Spirit Path Press.

_____. 2003. *The Clinical Practice of Chinese Medicine*. Stockbridge, Mass.: Spirit Path Press.

Matsumoto, Kiiko, and Stephen Birch. 1985. *Five Elements and Ten Stems*. Brookline, Mass.: Paradigm Publications.

Requena, Yves. 1989. *Character and Health: The Relation of Acupuncture and Psychology*. Brookline, MA: Paradigm Publications.

Ryle, Gilbert. 1949. *The Concept of Mind*. Chicago: University of Chicago Press.

Sivin, Nathan, ed. 1973. *Chinese Science: Explorations of an Ancient Tradition*. Cambridge, Mass.: Harvard University Press.

Willmont, Dennis. 1998. "The Evolution of Will, Destiny, and Wisdom." *Oriental Medical Journal* 7.3-4: 29-76.

Wiseman, Nigel. 1994. *Fundamentals of Chinese Medicine*. Brookline, Mass.: Paradigm Publications.

Chapter 3
Visions of the Body

The body is the key to understanding and transforming the self, be it for healing, long life, or immortality. It consists of the ongoing interchange of various forms of universal *qi*, identified as bodily energies and fluids. These are typically divided into yin and yang, depending on whether they are grosser or subtler and flow more on the surface or in the interior of the body.

The most basic yang force is personal *qi*. It constitutes health and sickness and determines how we move, eat, sleep, and function in the world. Flowing through meridians that have not been matched to anything in Western anatomy, it is the source of movement in and of the body, present in continuous circulation. Also, through breath, food, drink, physical contact, sexuality, and emotions, this *qi* is in constant exchange with the outside world. As noted earlier, it can be proper, well aligned, harmonious, right in amount and timing and activity, or wayward, heteropathic, misaligned, off track, and harmful.

The yin counterpart of personal *qi* is *xue*, often translated as "blood." It passes through veins that run deep in the body and includes various fluids known from Western anatomy, such as blood and lymph, but also carries internal life force and is considered the matrix of the mind. Problems in respect to *xue* tend to involve deficiencies or obstructions, presenting in paleness and lackluster, dry skin, or in sharp pains, tumors, cysts, and swellings.

Xue is closely connected to *qi*, often described as the wagon drawn by the horse of *qi*. Both are metabolized from the interaction of "grain-*qi*" (*guqi*, food) in the stomach and small intestine and "empty *qi*" (*kongqi*, air) in the lungs under the impact of the transformative power of heart-fire. This produces internal *qi*, which is further differentiated into the various bodily forces. This metabolism is the work of the triple heater (*sanjiao*), sometimes also called the triple burner. A uniquely Chinese entity, it is described in the *Yellow Emperor's Inner Classic* as providing a connection between heaven (upper heater), humanity (middle heater), and earth (lower heater). Over time the triple heater came to be associated with the aspects of the body cavity: thoracic, abdominal, and pelvic, i.e., the lungs, small intestine, and bladder. Commencing its function immediately after birth, the triple heater system takes the place of the integrated nourishment from primordial and mother *qi* in the womb and controls the transport, utilization, and excretion of the body's energies.

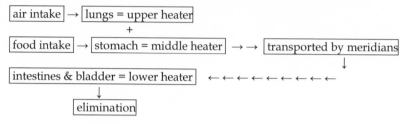

Fig. 5. The working of the triple heater

The triple heater is also responsible for the production of another yin-yang pair of energies, the protectors (*weiying*). They are forms of *qi* that pulsate through the body at different levels to defend and nurture it. *Wei* is yang in quality and commonly called protective or defensive *qi*. It moves next to the meridians and travels widely around the body, nourishing and strengthening the skin. It regulates the sweat glands, moistens the skin and hair, nourishes the tissues, and controls the opening and closing of the skin's pores. Its main job is to form a defense against harmful outside influences and pathogenic stress. It maintains the stability of the body, somewhat like the immune system in Western medicine.

Ying, the other protector in the body, is yin in nature and usually called constructive or nutritive *qi*. It is associated with the *xue*-blood and moves with it. It nourishes the muscles and the organs and ensures that the body's tissues remain strong. *Wei* and *ying* are a complementary pair, like *qi* and blood. They are characterized similarly in that their yin aspect is thicker and heavier and stays deep within the body, while its yang counterpart is thinner and lighter and moves at the surface of the body, interfacing with the outside world.

The same also holds true for the body fluids (*jinye*). They are defined as nutritive substances, formed when food in the digestive process is subjected to the functions of the stomach, spleen, lungs, and so on. Among them, *jin* are yang in nature. They appear as light, clear fluids that come to the body's surface due to internal processes. Examples include saliva (associated with the kidneys), tears (liver), sweat (heart), nasal mucus (lungs), and oral mucus (spleen). They lubricate the skin and the flesh. *Ye*, on the other hand, are yin. They are heavy, thick fluids diffused internally due to body movement, as for example lymph and internal mucus. They lubricate the joints and tendons, protect the brain, and fill the spine. The fluids, when produced in their appropriate amounts, serve as protectors and lubricants of the body. When they are deficient or excessive, however, they can be useful diagnostic tools. For example, a person with continuous dryness in the nose may well be suffering from chronic hay fever which affects his *qi*-flow even when it is not acute.

Functioning between these various yin and yang energies is *jing*, often translated as "essence." As Manfred Porkert in his *Theoretical Foundations of Chinese Medicine* defines it, *jing* is the indeterminate aspect of *qi* or *qi* in transition from one determinate form to another. A classic example is man's semen that carries life from the father to the child; another is the essence that the body takes from food during its assimilation. Neither yin nor yang, *jing* marks *qi* in transit, the raw fuel that drives the pulsating rhythm of the body's cellular reproduction. Governed by the kidneys and the phase water, it is also connected to the primordial *qi* that resides there and to the psychological power of will or determination. It is among the main sources of a person's charisma, sexual attraction, and sense of wholeness.

In its dominant form *jing* is sexual potency, that is, semen in men and menstrual blood in women. Both develop form of pure *qi* that sinks down from its center—the Ocean of *Qi* in the abdomen in men and the Cavern of *Qi* in the breast area in women—and becomes tangible in sexual sensations and fluids. Emitting *jing* from the body is seen as a major source of *qi*-loss which can cause physical weakness, lead to diseases, and precipitate early death. But even without excessive loss of *jing*, vital essence will diminish over a lifetime. Its rise and decline are understood as occurring in an eight-year cycle in males and a seven-year cycle in females. As the *Yellow Emperor's Inner Classic* says:

> When a girl is 7 years of age, the kidney *qi* [*jing*] becomes abundant. She begins to change her teeth and the hair grows longer. At 14, she begins to menstruate and is able to become pregnant. The movement of the great pulse is strong. The menses come regularly, and the girl is able to give birth.
>
> At age 21, the energy is steady, the last tooth has come out, and she is fully grown. When she reaches the age of 28, her tendons

and bones are strong, her hair has reached its full length, and her body is flourishing and fertile. At 35, her yang brightness pulse begins to slacken, her face begins to wrinkle, her hair starts falling out.

When she reaches the age of 42, the pulse of the three yang regions deteriorates in the upper part of her body, her entire face is wrinkled, and her hair turns gray. At age 49, she can no longer become pregnant, and the circulation of the great pulse is decreased. Her menstruation is exhausted, and the gates of blood are no longer open. Her body declines, and she is no longer able to bear children. (ch. 1)

To regulate and possibly slow down this process, there are various medical, longevity, and Daoist practices that control sexual energies and teach people to retain and strengthen their *jing*, even cause it to revert back to *qi* and thus renew life. They commonly involve both physical disciplines and meditation practices, allowing the *qi* to sink down and transform into *jing*, rendering it tangible as sexual arousal, but then preventing it from being emitted and instead reverting it back to *qi*.

Beyond the more tangible, fluid forms of *qi* in the body, there is also a pair of yin and yang energies that are more elusive and more psychological or spiritual in nature, yet are seen as forms of cosmic *qi*. They are spirit (*shen*) and numen (*ling*). Spirit is classified as yang and understood as the guiding vitality behind the various other forces. It is the active, organizing configurative force and transformative influence in the person; it connects him or her to heaven and original destiny. It manifests as individual consciousness and constitutes the individual's awareness and mental direction. Associated with the upper heater, it resides in the heart and is related to the mind and the emotions. It is an important cause of sickness, since much *qi*-exchange with the outside world happens through the emotions. Impossible to be perceived directly and physically, spirit is a vitalizing force that exerts transformative influence on all other aspects of the human being (Kaptchuk, *Web*, 58).

Numen is the yin counterpart of spirit. Largely ignored by practitioners in Communist China, it is sometimes translated as "soul" and designates the inherent spiritual self-nature of beings, the numinous power behind their physical presence. Supplementary to spirit, it is more internal and less obvious in interaction with the outside world, but appears in the names of five acupuncture points. It comes to the fore in death, when the remaining spiritual aspect of the person is called "numen." In fact, both spirit and numen are very much religious terms in traditional China. *Shen* also means "divine," god," and "ancestral spirit;" *ling* indicates "numinous," "ghostly," "soul," and "supernatural entity." Both can best be understood as the potential in human beings that works behind the scenes, either active and moving (spirit) or organizing and latent (numen).

Exercise: Review the classical symptoms of the common cold and examine how the different forms of body energies are affected by it. For example, feeling out of sorts: a lowering of spirit.

The body in Chinese health and long life practices, then, is the active combination of the various forms of *qi* and the inner organs as classified according to the five phases. These aspects of the body are never static or solitary, but exist in interaction and constant change. In Chinese cosmology, the body is further linked with the workings of the world and seen as a microcosmic replica of the natural and social world. As the *Book of the Master of Huainan* (*Huainanzi*), a Daoist collection of about 150 B.C.E., says:

> The roundness of the head is an image of heaven, the square shape of the feet matches the pattern of earth. Heaven has four seasons, five phases, nine directions, and 360 days. Human beings have four limbs, five inner organs, nine orifices, and 360 joints. Heaven has wind, rain, cold, and heat. Human beings have the actions of giving, taking, joy, and anger. The gall bladder corresponds to clouds, the lungs to breath, the liver to wind, the kidneys to rain, and the spleen to thunder. (ch. 7)

In expansion of this image, the body is also seen as a model for the way government functions, associating the heart with the ruler, the lungs with the civil administration, the liver with the military, and the gall with the judiciary. As the *Yellow Emperor's Inner Classic* says:

> The heart is the residence of the ruler; spirit and clarity originate here. The lungs are the residence of the high ministers of state; order and division originate here. The liver is the residence of the strategists; planning and organization originate here. The gall is residence of the judges; judgments and decisions originate here.
>
> The center of the breast is the residence of a special task-force; joy and pleasure originate here. The stomach is the residence of

the granary administration; the various kinds of taste originate here. The large intestine is the residence of the teachers of the Dao; development and transformations originate here. . . . The kidneys are the residence of the business men; activity and care originate here. (ch. 3)

In medieval Daoism, these natural and administrative models of the body are developed further to see the human body not only as a combination of natural patterns and energies but also as an inner sphere containing supernatural landscapes and divine beings. As a result, the body is described as a landscape with mountains and rivers, a divine and cosmic landscape, a paradise, a visible residence of the gods.

This is described in the *Yellow Court Scripture* (*Huangting jing*), a visualization manual from the fourth century C.E., and in a more recent visual depiction, the *Chart of Interior Passages* (*Neijing tu*). Here the celestial headquarters within is located in the head and matches the immortals' paradise of Mount Kunlun. It is depicted as a large, luscious mountain surrounded by a wide lake and covered with splendid palaces and wondrous orchards.

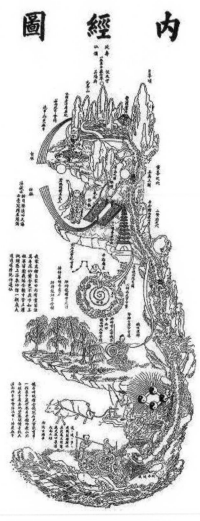

Between the eyes, which are the sun and the moon, one can move inside the head to the Hall of Light, one of nine palaces in the head. Best reached by passing through the deep, dark valley of the nose, it is guarded by the two high towers of

Fig. 6. The *Chart of Interior Passages*.

the ears. To attain entry one has to "beat the heavenly drum": with both palms covering the ears, snap the index and middle fingers to drum against the back of the skull.

Underneath the valley of the nose is a small lake, i.e., the mouth. This regulates the water level of the upper lake in the head and raises or lowers it as necessary. Crossing the mouth lake over its bridge (tongue) and moving further down, one reaches the twelve-storied tower of the throat, then comes to the Scarlet Palace (heart), the Yellow Court (spleen), the Imperial Granary (stomach), the Purple Chamber (gall), and various other starry palaces transposed into the body's depth. Going ever deeper, another cosmic region is reached, with another sun and moon (kidneys). Beneath them, the Ocean of *Qi* extends with another Mount Kunlun in its midst. Various divine beings, moreover, reside in the body, creating vitality and providing spiritual resources (Kohn, "Taoist Visions," 235).

The Daoist vision of the body as a network of celestial passageways and starry palaces closely overlaps with the medical understanding of the body as consisting of various aspects of *qi* and the phase-energetics of the five organs and six viscera. Many acupuncture points have Daoist connotations, and Chinese healing practices are at the root of Daoist practice. Without losing any aspect of the medical dynamics, this vision provides a more cosmic and spiritual dimension of the same basic understanding, allowing adepts to move beyond the physicality of their existence toward a greater, more spiritual realm, reaching out for the gods in the stars and thereby for the Dao at the center.

In contrast to this dynamic and spiritual vision of the body as an integrated whole and active part of the larger universe, the dominant Western understanding until very recently has tended to see the body as mere flesh, a material entity different from and opposed to the immortal soul, which alone belongs to God. The body is conceived as threatening and dangerous, full of unruly, ungovernable, and irrational passions. It has to be controlled at all costs, limited in its locations, excretions, and reproduction. Especially sexual energy, a mainstay of healing and long life in China, is seen as passion and the source of uncontrolled behavior, closely associated with evil. Thus there are the official norm of procreative monogamy in the West, the condemnation of relations with multiple partners, and the exultation of continence and celibacy.

Many Western ideas go back to ancient Greece, where moral virtue was associated with free men who regulated the public sphere and excluded women, adolescents, and slaves. For them, sexual pleasure threatened self-mastery, was closely regulated, and had no place in the public world. Christianity intensified this attitude toward the body, making it even more ascetic, demanding more control, and promoting the idea of the weak flesh that has to be subdued. A vision of reality emerged that was dualistic in nature, split between body and mind, desire and reason, world and God, Dionysos and Apollo. The body as flesh became a metaphor of the fallen man, original sin, and rejection by the deity. It was subdued to the point of total control and regulation, not only of the body but also of sexuality, and especially female sexuality. On a broader political and cultural level, this same urge to subdue and control then equaled a general ethic of world mastery (see Turner, *Body and Society*).

In the Enlightenment of the seventeenth century, medieval Christian lines of thinking were secularized and radicalized. An instrumental rationality in the form of science and technology was imposed on nature and social relations, just as through colonialism Christianity and Western culture came to dominate other cultures. Logic and goal-orientation superseded all aspects of emotionality. Control, seen as the power to be like the deity and ultimately aimed at the ability to create, became a central issue: control of the flesh through conquering sexuality and passions; control of the mind through systematic training, education, and political propaganda; control of nature through agriculture and industry, doing away with wilderness and wild life, and allowing nature to persist only in parks; control of the outer world by conquest of alien societies and the establishment of colonies; and control of all otherness though the increasing unification of world culture, the McDonaldization of society.

As part of this thrust toward control, the body was restricted more stringently through dietary practices and medical regimens, and the medical profession—in earlier ages not specialized but varied, not clinical but home-centered—became part of an effort at the total control of the world. It increasingly took over the place of the clergy, telling people what they could and could not do, and dominating the daily lives of ordinary folk. Religious notions of diet and asceticism were gradually replaced by secular medical perspectives. Where in earlier ages the key concern was with the interior body and its passions, in the nineteenth and early twentieth centuries people focused on the regulation of the exterior body with a new conception of domestic culture. Women were medically categorized as hysterical, reflecting male anxiety about the introduction of women into professional occupations. Antibiotics were discovered and proved effective to halt most infections, thus increasing the mechanical vision of the body and social control over it.

A totally different dimension in the Western understanding of the body came to the forefront in the late twentieth century. An increasingly consumer-based and consumer-oriented society no longer considered the body mere flesh and loosened the constraints of control. This society increasingly supported promiscuity and hedonism, encouraging people to try new things, buy more, and improve continuously. Credit and consumption became the key mainstays of culture, and the body was proclaimed a vehicle of pleasure. This, however, brought its own set of problems. Society, in order to be productive, still needs a disciplined workforce. Thus, today we have rules and ascetic propositions of body control, manifest in health clubs, diet fads, low-calorie drinks, nonfat foods, vitamin supplements, and generally visions of athletic beauty. At the same time, society also needs people to consume and buy more, and accordingly encourages them to pamper and enjoy themselves, giving free rein to their bodily desires—through nice meals, spa vacations, fancy clothes, electronic gadgets, sexual attractiveness, and so on.

The body in Western society has thus become a major battle ground between asceticism and hedonism, control and suppression versus letting go and unashamed display. It has become an ideal, a vision, a project that has to be pursued and made, refashioned by face-lifts, breast augmentations, diets, jogging, weight-lifting, massages, and so on. Yet despite its new image, the body has remained an object, a firm, solid, independent entity that needs to be shaped and molded. In that respect it has not changed despite the social and doctrinal transformations from antiquity through medieval Christianity and the Enlightenment to early capitalism. The body has never reached the position it has had in China traditionally—a fluid, ever changing network of energies and cosmic forces that we do not have but that we are.

> **Exercise:** Examine your own or a friend's lifestyle and body image in terms of asceticism and hedonism and find where choices reflect the current values of society. Give three examples.

As complementary medicine spreads, the pluralism already found in religion gradually becomes available in medicine. Slowly choices increase and the courts increasingly grant the rights of patients to choose or deny treatment. A new vision of the body, neither of asceticism and total control nor of consumerism and total indulgence, may emerge. In this cultural context the Chinese approach to health and long life is very important in that it helps us to see the body as an actively vibrating network of *qi* that participates actively in the larger oscillating universe. Its holistic view, key to a new level of integral, multifaceted medicine, allows us treat disorders as expressions of overall disharmony rather than isolated symptoms or malfunctions of specific parts. Medicine, rather than merely managing symptoms, comes to encourage the body to develop in a cosmic dimension, neither suppressing it nor glorifying its physicality.

Further Readings

Bynum, Caroline Walker. 1991. *Fragmentation and Redemption: Essays on Gender and the Human Body in Medieval Religion*. New York: Zone Books.

Feher, Michael, ed. 1989. *Fragments for a History of the Human Body*. New York: Urzone.

Fisher, Seymour. 1973. *Body Consciousness: You Are What You Feel*. Englewood Cliffs, N.J.: Prentice Hall.

Kohn, Livia. 1991. "Taoist Visions of the Body." *Journal of Chinese Philosophy* 18: 227-52.

Kuriyama, Shigehisa. 1999. *The Expressiveness of the Body and the Divergence of Greek and Chinese Medicine*. New York: Zone Books.

Laqueur, Thomas. 1990. *Making Sex: Body and Gender from the Greeks to Freud*. Cambridge, Mass.: Harvard University Press.

Law, Jane Marie. 1994. *Religious Reflections on the Human Body*. Bloomington: Indiana University Press.

Porkert, Manfred. 1974. *The Theoretical Foundations of Chinese Medicine*. Cambridge, Mass.: MIT Press.

Schipper, Kristofer M. 1994. *The Taoist Body*. Translated by Karen C. Duval. Berkeley: University of California Press.

Seem, Mark. 1989. *Body-Mind Energetics: Toward a Dynamic Model of Health*. Rochester, VT: Healing Arts Press.

Turner, Bryan S. 1984. *The Body and Society: Explorations in Social Theory*. Oxford: Basil Blackwell.

Chapter 4
Understanding the Mind

As the perspective of the body shifts toward greater openness and more fluidity, the understanding of the mind also has to undergo a major transition. The traditional Western vision, as noted earlier, is based on the Christian divide between pure spirit and impure matter, i.e., the polarization of a spirit that is eternal, divine, transcendent, and totally other and the body that is gross, transient, mundane, worldly, and physical. The body is seen as mere flesh and subjected to control, suppressed in favor of the spirit and the immortal soul. The mind is identified as rational thinking, the closest part to spirit and godliness within human beings, a force trained over and against the body.

The dualistic Western vision of human existence is formulated most explicitly in the works of the Renaissance thinker René Descartes, after whom it has been named the Cartesian model. He saw animals as machines that could not feel pain, but had a mechanical squeak reaction if you pinched them. Only human beings truly existed, because they were capable of thought. Thus, his most famous statement: "Cogito ergo sum." More than that, the only part truly alive and worth supporting in human beings is the *res cogitans*, the thinking, rational part of the mind. The Cartesian model established the superiority of mind over matter, above and beyond the ontological division of spirit and flesh as irreconcilable substances. This understanding led to scientific experiments and technological exploration, and, as noted above, goes together with visions of world mastery and the conquest of nature.

In the twentieth century, various new modes of looking at the body-mind phenomenon emerged, especially by the French philosophers Henri Bergson and Maurice Merleau-Ponty, who favored a more dynamic, process-based understanding. In addition, new developments in psychology began to overcome the mind-body split. Some represented a radical materialism and placed all emphasis on the body to see only learned behavioral responses, mediated by brain chemicals and neurotransmitters. Others, influenced by process philosophy and quantum physics, challenged this in favor of a more open-ended, interactive-field vision of body and mind (see Varela et al., *Embodied Mind*).

From the perspective of modern physics, the body is constantly vibrating and forms part of a universal pattern. The muscles and flesh are made from highly ordered, crystalline material, consisting of tiny atoms vibrating in groups along coiled molecules. The patterns are constant, rapid, and orderly. When subjected to the influence of a magnet or a needle, the field is modified and the whole pattern changes. The same also holds true for bones, which consist of vibrating patterns and changing energy fields — dissolving into the nothingness of pure oscillation when observed closely under the microscope.

The mind, then, is essentially the same as the body. There is no separation of consciousness from physical existence. Both are energy fields; they just vibrate at different speeds: 10^{22} Hz for the atomic nucleus, 10^{15} for the atom itself, 10^9 for molecules, and 10^3 for cells. Sensations in the body accordingly do not come from specific sense organs but arise through the fluctuation of different vibratory fields — all of which are immediately linked with consciousness in a non-local way, and in fact, *are* consciousness (see Targ and Katra, *Miracles of Mind*).

Consciousness, moreover, is unlimited and non-local, with powers beyond the range of the traditional, mechanical universe. Contemporary physicists and psychologists have recognized this fact, and numerous experiments have proven beyond all doubt that extrasensory perception (ESP) and subtle mental powers (*psi*) exist. They distinguish four different areas of their manifestation: telepathy, the clear understanding of another person's thoughts; clairvoyance, the vision of physical reality otherwise hidden; precognition, the knowledge of future conditions or events; and psycho kinesis, the ability to move physical objects with mental powers (see Tart et al., *Mind at Large*). While unexplained as to how they work exactly and how they can be activated or learned, these aspects of the human mind are powerful factors in the current rethinking of the body-mind continuum in Western culture.

> **Exercise:** Go to the web and find out more about current research on ESP and parapsychological powers. What are some of the latest theories on their functioning and activation? How can they influence healing?

The essential oneness of the body-mind and the inherent powers of thinking and perception have been central in faith healing and the laying-on of hands as practiced in many cultures. They also form a key aspect in East Asian efforts to heal diseases and help individuals fulfill their destiny. In Chinese thinking, the various aspects of human existence—body forces, forms of mentation, and psychological activities—are all different aspects of *qi*, vibrating at different speeds and manifesting at subtler or grosser levels. As a result, medical and Daoist texts do not show a separation of mental from bodily symptoms but take both as indications of disharmony. According to them, the word "mind" (*xin*) has two meanings: it is a general term for all the various aspects of consciousness and mental activity, and it is also a more specific term for the evaluation of the world in terms of good and bad, likes and dislikes, based on sensory stimuli, emotions, and classificatory schemes.

In this second sense, the mind is contrasted with the spirit (*shen*). Spirit is understood as the primordial, formless, and ever-changing force of life, which in connection with the physical body causes human beings to be alive. It occurs in its most concentrated form in the heart and ideally works through the mind in its more general sense to govern life perfectly. However, people get sidetracked through their involvement with sensory attractions and the pure spirit is transformed into an opinionated and limited mind through the senses and emotions. Confused and defiled, human beings need to be taught how to recover the primordial state. Both spirit and mind are associated with the inner organ of the heart, also called *xin*, and represent different aspects of consciousness—one evaluative and critical, essential for day-to-day survival in the ordinary world, the other flowing smoothly and open to all stimuli, the manifestation of the Dao within.

The spirit, moreover, is often matched with essence (*jing*), and the pair "spirit and essence" is used as a compound to describe the body-mind system. As part of essence, the mind is active in the blood (*xue*) and circulates along with it, but it is also concentrated in the storehouse of essence in the lower abdomen—the kidneys in medical discourse, the lower cinnabar or elixir field (*dantian*) in Daoism. By focusing their thoughts on this area, practitioners can gain peace and stability both in body and mind.

The mind is not simply spirit or essence, however, but as outlined in the *Yellow Emperor's Inner Classic* divides into five different forms, associated with the five inner organs:

> *Xue* is stored in the liver—the residence of the spirit soul.
> *Yingqi* is stored in the spleen—the residence of the intention.

> The pulse is stored in the heart — the residence of the spirit.
> Qi is stored in the lungs — the residence of the material soul.
> Essence is stored in the kidneys — the residence of the will. (ch. 2)

Each inner organ, therefore, has its own particular body fluid or form of *qi* and also its specific mental or psychological energy. They each transform and mutate into one another, according to the cycle of the five phases, so that *xue* is a transformation of constructive *qi*, and the pulse is another form of *qi*, closely related to the protective and constructive energies. As waves of the various energetic fluids move around the body, so the different aspects of the mind flow along all its parts, creating an integrated network of consciousness.

Among these different aspects, spirit is the most potent and most fundamental, associated with the heart, the leader of the organs and seat of the ruler (Ishida, "Body and Mind," 53). It is closely linked with two types of souls, sets of psychological forces that are described as spirit powers supporting the person yet working in opposite directions. The three spirit or cloud souls (*hun*) are yang in nature and relate to the liver. Envisioned as cultured officials, they guide humans toward the godlike and spiritual. The seven material or white souls (*po*) are yin in quality and connect to the lungs. Depicted as half-demons, they support people in their instinctual and animal aspects.

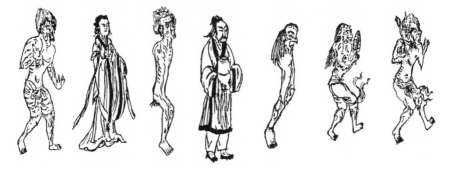

Fig. 7. The seven material souls.

Exercise: Think of some instincts and egotistic patterns that might be associated with the material souls. Why are they necessary for human survival? What are possible benefits of having them? How do they turn into negative forces? Are they still necessary today?

Beyond the souls, there are two further mental forces, called will (*zhi*; yin) and intention (*yi*; yang) which function in close relation to the kidneys and spleen. They are specific aspects of the mind, i.e., the general power of thinking and planning in the intention and the more focused determination directed toward a specific object found in the will. All these aspects of the mind are in constant interaction and change, so that consciousness as the integrated flux of various forces and energies.

Essence and spirit, then, are the most primordial aspects of the mind as it is received from heaven and earth. The two kinds of souls are its moving and active dimensions that determine human attitudes, thoughts, and desires, while will and intention are its concrete everyday functions. In general, the yin aspects are more body-oriented, material, and linked with earth, while the yang aspects are more spirit-oriented, ethereal, and linked with heaven. Thus, the intention can be described as the thinking mind, while the will is the thinking body. The entirety of both, however different they may be in vibrational frequency and orientation, makes up human consciousness.

The outward manifestations of these inner functions are the emotions. They are each associated with specific organs: anger with the liver, excessive joy or hatred with the heart, worry with the spleen, sadness with the lungs, and fear with the kidneys. They are judged negatively, since they are seen as excesses of natural *qi*-patterns and reactions that go beyond what is suitable in the transformation of the phases. For example, it is entirely appropriate to feel courage and engage in new ventures in the spring (liver); to be enthusiastic and joyful in the summer (heart); to plan ahead and think about the coming winter in late summer (spleen); to be thoughtful and pensive in the decline of the seasons in the fall (lungs); and to exercise caution when things are icy and frozen in winter (kidneys).

While these mental attitudes are perfectly in line with the seasonal cycle of nature and form a natural expression of the *qi* of the inner organs, the emotions are their excesses—fear is caution gone haywire, anger is enthusiasm turned into impatience and aggression. They lead to a depletion of *qi* in their respective organs, creating energetic disharmony which in turn increases the intensity of the emotion. Then the emotion may turn on itself and multiply. For example, reacting to fear with fear, a person may become paranoid, sly and secretive, lying to others and only intent on self-interest. Similarly, someone full of anger may feel angry at being so aggressive and become deeply resentful of himself and others, seething inside while trying to manipulate people around him.

These negative patterns, moreover, are not limited to one emotion or organ. Once one is affected, the disharmony spills over to the next through the cycle of the five phases, and negative feelings are compounded. Thus fear and anger (kidneys and liver) are connected, and so are sadness and hatred (lungs and heart). As the *Yellow Emperor's Inner Classic* says:

> When the *qi* of the liver is too empty there is fear [kidney emotion]; when it is too full, there is anger [liver emotion]. . . .
> When the *qi* of the heart is too empty there is sorrow [lung emotion]; when it is too full there is excessive joy [heart emotion]. (ch. 3)

The emotions are closely related to the *qi*-body and can serve either as diagnostic *qi*-flow symptoms or as a way to better health. They are central in regulating body movements, food intake, breathing, and mental clarity. Perception, respiration, excretion, and all the various physical and psychological functions relating to the body's orifices, are governed by the mental functions, psychological forces, and emotions, as they reside in the five organs and appear in different forms.

The Chinese understanding, therefore, does not locate the mind in one major center, such as the brain or the heart, but sees it as flowing and flexible (see Ishida, "Body and Mind"). The mind is where the intention is and where the spirit resides. It can be either wide open and flowing everywhere or concentrated in one specific body part. For example, when someone is absorbed in reading or listening or some other activity, the mind is focused there to the exclusion of all else. However, if the mind is guided to move smoothly around the body and comes to fill more of it, higher states of mental awareness result. The actively flowing mind, achieved in meditative exercises of guided breathing and circulated intention, leads to greater mental purity. This in turn can overflow to the outside and manifest in a glowing facial complexion and a stronger *qi*-quality in exchange with others. People who have attained a high level of the flowing mind are considered beautiful and charismatic, energized and "spirited." Further levels of the pervasive awareness of mind and *qi* can also lead to cosmic consciousness, not unlike the "peak-experiences" described in Western psychology or even the mystical experiences of different religions. Reaching this state as understood in the Chinese system, aside from the mental freedom, also means a greater degree of physical integration; it helps to assure health and longevity and may even lead to immortality.

Daoism picks up on this vision and states that, as the mind is consciously guided around the body and the person observes five basic precepts against violent actions, the emotions are purified not only from their excess to a suitable level of appropriate reaction but into virtues. The virtues in this system are adapted from the Confucian canon, lauded already by Confucius (551-479 B.C.E.) and Mencius (372-289 B.C.E.) as the key factors in creating a well-integrated individual and harmonious society. The different emotions, then, are transformed as follows:

phase	organ	precept	emotion	appropriate	virtue
wood	liver	no killing	anger frustration	assertion	benevolence compassion
fire	heart	no licentiousness	excessive joy hatred	enthusiasm	propriety respect
earth	spleen	no lying	worry resentment	planning	reciprocity empathy
metal	lungs	no intoxication	sadness cruelty	thoughtfulness	righteousness
water	kidneys	no stealing	fear loneliness	caution	wisdom care, trust

Both self-cultivation practices and meditations are used to overcome excessive emotions and negative *qi*-patterns. Gradually, as people relax and their *qi* begins to flow more smoothly, they replace strong emotions with appropriate reactions—a goal both in medical and longevity practice. From here practitioners can develop further toward a sense of harmony with the Dao and wholeness in themselves, opening to others and becoming more altruistic. As they grow in compassion, respect, and care, they attain the Confucian virtues and realize a more altruistic and universally-minded mode of being (Kohn, *Cosmos and Community*, 32).

Daoist practice suggests that adepts begin with one emotion which stands out as dominant and which can be felt and observed most clearly. This may mean visualizing oneself in an excess of the emotion to see how ludicrous its nature is, then understanding its underlying patterns and transforming it. From there, the others can be unraveled, because the emotions, following the productive cycle of the five phases, tend to move from one into the next. Anger leads to hatred, hatred to resentment, resentment to cruelty, cruelty to fear, and fear again to anger. The latter connection is also well known in Western psychology, where anger is commonly seen as a symptom of suppressed pain and fear.

In the same way, when even one virtue is embraced, the productive cycle will take over and the others will come to grow. Thus, compassion leads to respect, respect demands honesty, honesty brings about thoughtfulness, thoughtfulness leads to gentleness, and gentleness opens the doors to compassion. And, of course, true virtue begins at home, so practitioners are advised to relax in their demands on themselves first, becoming comfortable in who and what they are, then extend their well-being into the world.

The most central virtue of all is honesty, associated with the phase earth, the direction of the center, and the spleen and stomach in the body. Once honesty is found and one has faith in oneself, one can develop trust in other people and begin to care for them, enhancing all the virtues.

> **Exercise:** Think of an emotion that is strong in your life. Identify it in terms of the five phases and see how it relates to other emotions and how you could transform it into an appropriate reaction or even a virtue. What mental reorientation would be necessary?

Beyond the virtues, Daoists also believe in the presence of divine agents in the body. Among them are most prominently the Three Ones and the Three Corpses or Deathbringers. The Three Ones, yang in nature, are pure deities of the Dao who, through proper meditation, come to reside in the cinnabar fields in head, chest, and abdomen. They are an immediate manifestation of pure primordial *qi* and originally reside in heaven. Visualized according to sacred manuals and called down to be activated in the adept's body, they greatly benefit his or her life, bestowing divine powers of good fortune, long life, and immortality.

Their yin counterparts are the Three Deathbringers, a mixture of demons and parasites who reside in the head, chest, and abdomen, assisted by a group known as the Nine Worms. Together they incite the person to engage in excessive emotions, commit bad deeds, and fall ill. After the death of the host, when the various souls have been sent off to their respective realms of yin and yang, the Deathbringers remain with the corpse and gorge themselves on its blood, bones, and muscles. Having partaken of the human body, they are able to assume its former shape and appear as ghosts, feasting further on offerings laid out for the dead. They have thus a vested interest in bringing a person to death quickly and without mercy.

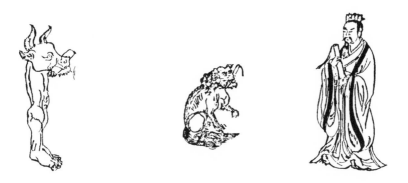

Fig. 8. The Three Deathbringers

Measures against them include virtuous behavior and emotional control as well as continued meditation on the Three Ones, who ideally will replace them and eventually make the person immortal. For those who lack saintly virtue, there are more physical countermeasures, such as a vigil on the night, once every two months (still practiced also in Japan), when the Three Deathbringers ascend to heaven to report to the celestial administration. They can only leave the body when the person is asleep and, without proper directives for destruction from above, will be helpless and disoriented and eventually will die. For people who cannot stay awake long enough or lack moral purity, herbs and medicines as well as certain taboos keep the Three Deathbringers from doing too much harm. While these remedies will not eradicate the Deathbringers and people may still die from their activities, these practices at least hamper them in their ways, and one can breathe a little easier (see Kohn, "Kôshin").

Similar measures can also be applied to demonic forces invading the body, a major cause of disease in ancient China. In fact, Paul Unschuld has suggested that the practice of acupuncture goes back to the stabbing of invasive demons with miniature lancets, and many medical textbooks contain treatments for possession. Possession can be described as the taking-over of an individual's function by hostile outside forces, demons or energetic imbalances that invade the body, or by inner powers turned harmful, such as the false ego that makes strong demands on the person. As Lonny Jarrett points out, people become vulnerable when their immunity is compromised because of poor living habits or receiving a major shock. Possessed patients tend to be so stuck in one form of thinking or emotion that there is no room for spontaneity, freedom, or flexibility. In these patients, there seems to be only darkness, the inner light of the true self being completely obscured. The patient tends to refuse direct eye contact but may well be aware of the condition, stating that "I don't quite feel like myself." Treatment involves specific spirit points as well as healing herbs which open and strengthen the person's qi-flow, so that the mind is not longer stuck at one point and the energetic system can eliminate the intruder (*Clinical Practice*, ch. 3).

The mind in Chinese culture is thus a complex phenomenon that consists of various mental forces and spiritual agents of yin and yang nature associated with the five inner organs and three cinnabar fields. Again, the emphasis is on qi-flow and the smoothness and balance of all internal forces.

Further Readings

Chia, Mantak, and Manewan Chia. 1989. *Fusion of the Five Elements: Basic and Advanced Methods for Transforming Negative Emotion into Positive Virtue.* Huntington, NY: Healing Tao Books.

Ishida, Hidemi. 1989. "Body and Mind: The Chinese Perspective." In *Daoist Meditation and Longevity Techniques*, edited by Livia Kohn, 41-70. Ann Arbor: University of Michigan, Center for Chinese Studies Publications.

Jarrett, Lonny S. 2003. *The Clinical Practice of Chinese Medicine.* Stockbridge, Mass.: Spirit Path Press.

Kohn, Livia. 1995. "Kôshin: A Taoist Cult in Japan. Part II: Historical Development." *Japanese Religions* 20.1: 34-55.

_____. 2004. *Cosmos and Community: The Ethical Dimension of Daoism.* Cambridge, Mass.: Three Pines Press.

Sivin, Nathan. 1995. "Emotional Encounter Therapy." In *Medicine, Philosophy and Religion in Ancient China.* Aldershot, U.K.: Variorum.

Targ, Russell, and Jane Katra. 1999. *Miracles of Mind: Exploring Nonlocal Consciousness and Spiritual Healing.* Novato, Calif.: New World Library.

Tart, Charles T., Harold E. Puthoff, and Russell Targ, eds. 1979. *Mind at Large.* New York: Praeger.

Unschuld, Paul U. 1985. *Medicine in China: A History of Ideas.* Berkeley: University of California Press.

Varela, Francisco, Evan Thompson, and Eleanor Rosch. 1991. *The Embodied Mind: Cognitive Science and Human Experience.* Cambridge, Mass.: MIT Press.

Chapter 5

The Meridian System

To access the various functions of *qi* in body and mind, practitioners regulate the flow of *qi* as it courses through the energy lines of the body, known as meridians (*jingluo*). Meridians are invisible channels of *qi*-circulation that connect the inner organs with the hands and feet and provide communication between the upper and lower body, interior and exterior. Flowing through them, *qi* moistens the bones and tendons, provides nutrition to the joints, and balances yin and yang.

There are twelve main meridians, grown from originally eleven—related to the five yin and five yang organs plus the triple heater. These were already listed in early Han manuscripts and expanded to twelve when a sixth yin-meridian, that of the pericardium, was added for symmetry in the early centuries C.E. The six yin meridians move essential *qi*, connect to spirit and souls, and are a function of overall health. They can be full or empty. The six yang meridians process active *qi* and run closer to the surface than their yin counterparts. They digest food, transmit fluids, and can be replete or exhausted due to pathological nutritional conditions. When their *qi* is excessive, there will be swelling and heat along the meridians; when their *qi* is deficient, chills and shivers appear. The twelve main meridians are as follows:

phase	yin merid	yang merid.	phase	yin meridian	yang meridian
wood	liver	gallbladder	metal	lungs	lg. intestine
fire	heart	sm. intestine	water	kidneys	bladder
earth	spleen	stomach	fire	pericardium	triple heater

The meridians are connected to the organs and like them are not solid, firm entities or aggregate carriers, but represent a fabric of functional manifestations. They are symbols associated with a wealth of body functions and cosmological phenomena and may be described as a bodily substratum of vague material and spatial contours. Their main purpose is to move *qi*; they are invisible yet tangible lines of communication, each associated with a particular activity or bodily function:

gallbladder: detoxification	liver: storage, distribution
small intestine: assimilation	heart: meaning, emotions

51

stomach: food intake	spleen: digestion
large intestine: *qi* elimination	lungs: *qi* intake
bladder: purification	kidneys: movement
triple heater: protection	pericardium: circulation

There are two complete sets of meridians in the body, one on the right and one on the left. They are not isolated but connect in several intricate networks, and are commonly described in the order of an energetic system that alternates yin and yang and hands and feet. The order is hand-hand, foot-foot, plus yin-yang yang-yin.

That is, all yin meridians either begin or end in the chest, while all yang meridians either begin or end in the head. They alternate between upward and downward movements, and go to or from either hand or foot. Typically yin meridians move down the arms and up the legs, while yang meridians move up the arms and down the legs.

Yin meridians run on the inner (medial) side of the extremities, while yang meridians follow paths on their outer (lateral) side. The complete pattern looks as follows (www.lieske.com; www.tcm-central.com):

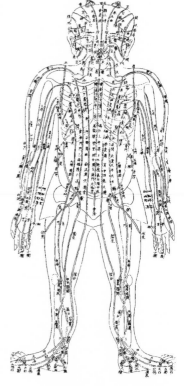

Fig. 9. The meridians in the body.

chest	yin	yang	head
to hand	1. lungs	2. large intestine	from hand
from foot	4. spleen	3. stomach	to foot
to hand	5. heart	6. small intestine	from hand
from foot	8. kidneys	7. bladder	to foot
to hand	9. pericardium	10. triple heater	from hand
from foot	12. liver	11. gallbladder	to foot

Exercise: Examine the tables on the previous pages to determine how the *qi*-flow in the meridians relates to the different cycles of the five phases (productive, controlling). Does it imitate one or the other?

The network begins with the lung meridian, characterized as yin. It starts in the chest (lungs), moves through the armpit and along the inner side of the arm, and ends at the thumb of the hand. It has 11 acupuncture points (*tsubo* in Japanese), that is, spots where the meridian comes closest to the surface and can be accessed by needles, heat, or finger pressure. The lung meridian is treated for symptoms of colds and cough, such as chills, asthma, wheezing, a weak voice, night sweats, and shortness of breath, but it can also be helpful in cases of shoulder and back pain. Important points for these symptoms include Central Prefecture (Zhongfu; Lu-1),[1] located in front of the armpit, and Inch Marsh (Chize; Lu-5) in the inner elbow (see www.yinyanghouse.com).

From the last point of the lung meridian at the thumb, the energetic network connects to its yang counterpart, the large intestine meridian. It begins at the index finger at Merchant Yang (Shangyang; LI-1), flows along the outside of the arm across the shoulder, neck, and upper lip to the nose, where it ends at the side of the nostril. One branch continues into the torso to the large intestine. Symptoms treated are toothache, nasal dryness, nosebleed, stiff shoulders, shivers, swellings in the arms or the face, as well as abdominal pains. The large intestine meridian has twenty points, the most popular among which is Meeting Valley (Hegu; LI-4,), in the junction between thumb and index finger. Also known as the "endorphin point," it is used for all kinds of ailments, from headaches through nausea to depression and stress. Its ending point, Smell Receptor (Yangxiang; LI-20) on the side of the nostril is used particularly to relieve stuffy noses.

Connecting from here to another yang channel, *qi* flows into the stomach meridian. It begins below the pupils at Producing Tears (Chengli; St-1) and passes the corner of the eye, the upper gums, lips, lower jaw, ears and forehead, then moves downward through the throat, chest, stomach, groin, and along the outside of the legs. It ends at the foot at Passing Open (Litui; St-45), on the medial side of the second toe. It is used to treat abdominal chills and distention, various intestinal problems, colds and

---

[1] The numbering of points and use of an appropriate abbreviation for the meridian is a Western contribution to Chinese medicine. It was first practiced by the French in the early twentieth century.

sneezes, a red complexion, and an aversion to people. Main points for this include Heavenly Pivot (Tianshu; St-25), two inches besides the navel[2] and Foot Third Mile (Zusanli; St-36), three inches below the knee. St-7, known as Lower Gate (Xiaguan) is on the side of the ear and helps with toothache and ear problems (see www.acuxo.com).

Linking to the yin counterpart of the stomach meridian, the flow of *qi* continues in the spleen meridian. It begins at White Yin (Yinbai; Sp-1) on the medial side of the big toe and passes over the instep, the inner side of leg, abdomen, and the chest to end at Great Embrace (Dabao; Sp-21) at the thorax. Used for digestive and gynecological problems, including diarrhea, nausea, the urge to vomit after eating, as well as menstrual cramps and irregularities, popular points include Three Yin Interchange (Sanyin jiao; Sp-6), three inches above the ankle and, especially for menstrual problems, Ocean of Blood (Xuehai; Sp-10), two inches above the knee. Other points can also help with motor problems, insomnia, chronic fatigue, lymph problems, cold limbs, asthma, chest pain, and swelling and pains at the root of the tongue.

The *qi*-flow then moves into the next yin meridian, that of the heart. Beginning at Ultimate Source (Jiyuan; He-1) at the armpit and with an internal branch connecting to the heart, it passes through the chest and lungs, moves along the side of the throat and through the inner side of arm. The heart meridian ends at Lesser Rise (Shaochong; Ht-9) on the inner corner of the tip of the little finger. Applications include chest pain, dizziness, dim eyesight, and dry throat, but also problems with the arms and hands and more psychological symptoms, such as emotional distress, depression, insomnia. The most important point for the latter is Spirit Gate (Shenmen; Ht-7), which is needled only with great caution—just as Chinese physicians tend to be reluctant to treat the heart meridian directly, instead using its lesser version, the pericardium.

At the little finger, at Lesser Marsh (Shaoze; SI-1) on the outside nail, begins the heart meridian's yang counterpart, the small intestine meridian. It runs along the outside of the hand, arm, shoulder, and upper back, then moves up the neck to the cheek and around the corner of the eye to end at the ear, at the Hearing Palace (Tinggong; SI-19). An internal

---

[2] The idea of inches in this system is matched to the size of the person's body. One inch (*cun*) is the length of the upper segment of the thumb or that of the central segment of the middle finger. The location of the points is measured in internal relation to the person. For images, go to www.tcmstudent.com/cunmeasure.shtml.

branch splits off at the clavicle to go through the esophagus and the stomach to the small intestine. Its points treat pain in the shoulders and upper arms, headaches, sore throat, bad hearing, and dim eyesight. Important points for these include Back Stream (Houchi; SI-3) on the pinky side of the palm and Yang Valley (Yanggu; SI-5) at the wrist.

Connecting from here to yet another yang meridian, the *qi*-flow moves into the bladder channel. The longest meridian, it begins at Pure Brightness (Jingming; Bl-1) at the inner corner of the eye and passes across the forehead, over the top of the skull, down the neck and over the shoulders to along the back. Here it runs parallel to the spine in two columns. Reaching the lower back, it moves across the buttocks and continues along the posterior thigh, passing the knees and calves to end on the outside of the foot, at the outer tip of the little toe. It has a total of sixty-seven points and is used for a variety of symptoms, including headaches, eye pressure, dim eyesight, flow of tears, clogged nose, stiff neck, back pain, stiff hips and knees, and hemorrhoids. Important points are Heavenly Pillar (Tianzhu; Bl-10) at the upper neck for head and eye trouble; Kidney Point (Shenshu; Bl-23) in the mid-back to enhance determination; and Command Center (Weizhong; Bl-40) at the back of the knee for back and leg pains as well as cramps. Open Valley (Tonggu; Bl-60) on the ankle, moreover, is known as the "aspirin point" and used for all sorts of ailments.

Beginning at the foot, more specifically at Bubbling Well (Yongquan; Ki-1) in the center of the sole, the kidney meridian is the yin counterpart of the bladder channel. It runs through the instep, circles around the medial ankle, moves up the inner leg and through the abdomen to the chest. It has twenty-seven points, used to treat lower back pain, ringing in the ears, anxiety, chills, gasping breath, dim eyesight, cold, chest pains, and pain in the feet. Linked with the kidneys and thus with sexual energy, it can also help with reproductive problems, for which notably Great Flow (Taixi; Ki-3) behind and above the ankle bone is used. A point that nurtures the heart, moreover, is Heart Pit Point (Huangshu; Ki-16) in the upper abdomen.

The next yin meridian is that of the pericardium or heart protector, abbreviated PC or HP. It begins next to the nipples and passes through the chest, armpits, and inner arm to end at the middle finger. It has nine points that are used to treat accelerated heart beat, compulsive laughter, flushed face, depression, hot flashes, depression, and burning in palms. Most important are Inner Gate (Neiguan; PC-6), located two inches above the wrist and helpful for stomach and chest problems as well as anxiety and memory enhancement. Labor Palace (Laogong; PC 8) in the center of the palm is a key gateway of *qi* and essential in Qigong practice and for external *qi*-healing.

The yang counterpart of the pericardium is the triple heater. Its meridian begins at the tip of the ring finger, passes along the outer arm, elbow, shoulder, chest, and throat to the side of face, where it circles the ear and ends at the cheek. It has twenty-three points and treats sore throat, deafness, ear trouble, sudden heat, facial swellings, and abdominal discomforts. An important point for fevers and chills is Outer Pass (Waiguan; TH-5), about two inches above the wrist.

The last pair of meridians are the gallbladder and the liver. The gallbladder, a yang channel that connects to the triple heater, begins at the outer corner of the eye and passes in a crisscross pattern over the side of head and the ears. It then moves through the shoulders, chest, and gallbladder, to reach the abdomen and hips. From here it goes on along the outer side of the leg and across the ankle and foot to end at the outer tip of the fourth toe. Its forty-four points treat emaciation, digestive problems, leg trouble, fevers and chills, eye pain, muscular tension, thigh and knee problems, and chest pain. In addition, Wind Pond (Fengchi; Gb-20) at the base of skull and Shoulder Well (Jianjing; Gb-21) are helpful for stiff shoulders, neck pain, and blurred vision, while Jumping Circle (Huantiao; Gb-30) at the hip is good for back and hip pain, and Yang Mound Spring (Yangling quan; Gb-34) below the knee enhances decision making and mental clarity.

Concluding the set of the twelve main meridians is the liver channel, the yin partner of the gallbladder. It begins at the tip of the big toe, on the side towards the second toe. From here it moves up the foot to the inner side of the leg, crosses the pubic region, lower abdomen, liver, and lungs to end in the rib cage, from where the *qi*-flow connects to the lungs and begins the whole cycle all over again. An internal branch ends at the liver. Its fourteen points treat depression, bad temper, painful chest, menstrual irregularities, blurred vision, joint pains, headaches, diarrhea, vomiting, digestive troubles, stiffness of hips, genital diseases, and the inability to urinate. Its most important point is Too Fast (Taichong; Li-3) on the top of the foot near the ankle. It is a strong point for moving *qi* and helps with numerous ailments, including headaches and dizziness.

Exercise: Pick five acupuncture points among the ones mentioned and locate them on your own body and/or the body of a friend. Find the area indicated, then locate the point by identifying a spot that is sensitive and slightly sore.

The *qi*-flow marked by the meridians in this order is not only a theoretical framework that creates a network and helps with memorization. It is actively present in the body and most obvious during specific times in the course of the day. The day is divided into twelve two-hour periods, and each meridian is believed to be dominant during one of them. If a particular weakness or pain appears during one of these hours, the respective meridian may have an imbalance. Also, treatment during these times is optimal and the meridian's functions are best enhanced then. The times are (see www.tcm.edu):

1. lungs	3-5 am	7. bladder	3-5 p.m.
2. large intestine	5-7 am	8. kidneys	5-7 p.m.
3. stomach	7-9 am	9. pericardium	7-9 p.m.
4. spleen	9-11 am	10. triple heater	9-11 p.m.
5. heart	11-1 p.m.	11. gallbladder	11-1 am
6. small intestine	1-3 p.m.	12. liver	1-3 am

Each meridian, moreover, is associated—through its organ's connection with the five phases—with a set of particular phenomena, including bodily aspects, such as types of voice and tissues, but also more generally cosmological things, including colors, tastes, animals, musical instruments, planets, and so on.

The bodily correspondences are:

organ1	body 1	body2	liquid	sound	sense	smell	taste	emotion
lungs	skin	body hair	mucus	weep	smell	raw	spicy	sadness
spleen	flesh	skin tone	saliva	sing	touch	fragrant	sweet	worry
heart	pulse	face color	sweat	laugh	taste	burnt	bitter	exc. joy
kidneys	bones	head hair	urine	moan	hear	putrid	salty	fear
liver	nerves	nails	tears	shout	see	rancid	sour	anger

More cosmologically, they are:

organ1	phase	color	season	planet	species	grain	music	direction
lungs	metal	white	fall	Venus	shell	rice	lithophone	west
spleen	earth	yellow	late sum.	Saturn	naked	millet	drums	center
heart	fire	red	summer	Mars	feathery	millet	reeds	south
kidneys	water	black	winter	Mercury	scaly	soy	zither	north
liver	wood	green	spring	Jupiter	furry	wheat	lute	east

These correspondences link the different aspects of the body and the universe into an integrated network, each part expressing the unity at the foundation of all. This unity means that the parts are ultimately one so that, for example, skin, lungs, white, and west do not match each other but *are* each other, expressed in the variable media of the world.

In practice, the correspondences mean that the physician looks at the functioning of the meridian not only on the basis of specific methods of diagnosis, but also in the context of the patient's overall lifestyle and physical presentation. For example, someone with excessive *qi*-flow in the spleen will tend to worry and often be involved in a profession that demands a lot of thinking. He or she will tend to have a sweet tooth, like to sing, enjoy late summer, prefer yellow, beige, and brown colors, and among musical instruments favor the drum. All the various tendencies of the individual are thus part of the overall picture of the diagnosis, not limiting either analysis or treatment to one single aspect.

In addition to the twelve main meridians there are various other sets of channels through the body, such as the twelve transverse channels which run horizontally through the body and connect the main meridians; the twelve tendon-muscular conduits which follow basically the same course as the main meridians but pass more superficially through the tissue and have no relationship with the inner organs; and the eight extraordinary or unpaired vessels, which are pre-organ functional containers of primordial *qi* and serve both in medical and spiritual practice. Called vessels (*mai*) rather than meridians (*luo*), they can be divided into two major groups of four, one set that is present in the body but does not get used very much in clinical and spiritual practice, and another that is rather important. The four less important vessels are:

> 1. Yin Activation Vessel (*yinqiao mai*). It begins at the ankle, the second point of the kidney meridian, and runs along the inner side of the leg and the center of the abdomen to the face, where it ends at the corner of the eyes, at the first point of the bladder meridian. Considered an offshoot of the kidney meridian, it exerts an influence on the *qi*-flow along this line and helps to tone leg muscles.

> 2. Yang Activation Vessel (*yangqiao mai*). It runs from the ankle along the outside of the legs and sides of the torso to the face, where it passes along the side of the eyes and ends at the ear. An offshoot of the bladder meridian, it influences the lateral aspect of the legs, back, neck, head, and eyes.

3. Yin Maintenance Vessel (*yinwei mai*). It runs from the central abdomen through the chest area to the throat, ending at the chin. It influences the chest and the heart, tonifies the blood, and connects all the various yin channels.

4. Yang Maintenance Vessel (*yangwei mai*). It begins at the outside edge of the foot slightly below the ankle, runs along the back of the legs, torso, and head, and ends at the neck. It connects all the yang channels and influences the lateral aspect of the legs, the sides of the body, neck, and head, as well as the ears.

The more important extraordinary vessels include three vertical and one horizontal line of *qi*. The horizontal line is known as the Belt Vessel (*daimai*). It runs around the abdomen a few inches below the navel, connecting the Ocean of *Qi* point in the front with the Gate of Destiny point in the back and linking both the vertical meridians and the major storehouses of *qi* and *jing*.

The other three extraordinary vessels are vertical lines through the torso, which link the pelvic floor with the head. The Penetrating Vessel (*chongmai*) runs right through the center. It begins at the perineum, a small cluster of muscles located between the anus and the genital organs, and reaches to the crown of the head, to a point known as Hundred Meeting (Baihui; GV-20). It connects the kidneys and stomach, as well as the various centers of *qi* in the body, and is considered the main conduit of primordial *qi*. Used medically for gynecological problems, its main application is in meditative and religious practices, whose adepts send their intention through it into the depth of their cinnabar fields and thus open their centers and connect to higher levels.

Next are the Conception Vessel (yin) and the Governing Vessel (yang), which run along the front and back of the torso respectively, reaching from the pelvic floor to the head. They are of great importance both in healing and religion, serving to mix *qi* and blood and to guide the *qi* along the major centers of the body.

The Conception Vessel (*renmai*) begins at Meeting of Yin (Huiyin; CV-1) at the perineum, passes through the front of the body along its central line, and ends at the mouth. A carrier and major supporter of yin *qi*, it has many medical applications. Its lower points are urogenital; its middle points are digestive; and its upper points are thoracic. Deficient *qi* in the Conception Vessel may be indicated by itchy skin. Together with the spleen meridian, it controls pregnancy and menstruation. It can be activated to treat asthma, coughs, dyspepsia, eczema, eye problems, hernia, influenza, laryngitis, and others. Among its twenty-four points, most important are Ocean of Qi (Qihai; CV-6) in the lower abdomen, Spirit Tower (Shenque; CV-8) at the navel, and Ocean of Tranquility (Jinghai; CV-17) at the center of the chest. They also tend to have a psychological impact. Two further points on this channel that are important in Daoist practice are Central Court (Zhongting; CV-16,) which matches the solar plexus, and Purple Palace (Zigong; CV-18), which matches the heart.

The Governing Vessel (*dumai*) also begins at Extended Strength (Changqiang; HV-1) at the coccyx , then passes along the back of the body following the spine, moves across the top of the head, and ends inside the mouth at the upper gums. It transports and aids yang-*qi*; its points connect to other channels and the various inner organs. It is needled in cases of runny eyes, neck pain, hernia, lumbago, sterility, urine retention, and hemorrhoids. Its twenty-eight points include also the more spiritual points Gate of Destiny (Mingmen; GV-4) at the 2nd-3rd lumbar vertebrae, Numinous Terrace (Lingtai; GV-10) at the 6th thoracic vertebra, as well as the Jade Pillow (Yuchen; GV-17) at the back of the skull which is needled for headaches and tension.

The two meridians connect at the mouth, with Fluid Receptacle (Chengjiang; CV-24) located at the lower lip and Gum Intersection (Yinjiao; GV-28) found at the upper gums. They also both continue internally, descending back to the pelvic floor and forming a continuous, intricate inner loop. Rather than using this path, however, adepts tend to activate them as one straight circle of *qi*-flow. They place the tongue at the roof of the mouth as a bridge between the meridians, then inhale deeply into the abdomen to enhance their Ocean of Qi or lower cinnabar field. From there, they breathe out, envisioning their *qi* flowing downward to the pelvic floor and reaching the perineum.

Focusing on the coccyx (GV-1), they inhale the *qi* up along the spine, passing through all the various points along the Governing Vessel. At Great Hammer (Dazhui; GV-15) below the neck, they begin to exhale, carrying the *qi* further up along the back of the skull, across Hundred Meeting (Baihui; GV-20), along the forehead and to the nostrils. From here they inhale again, envisioning the *qi* flowing down along the Conception Vessel and through the Ocean of Qi into the pelvic floor, thus establishing a cycle of *qi* throughout the torso.

This integrated *qi*-flow is known as the "microcosmic orbit" and is commonly used in Qigong to establish a *qi*-flow before physical movements and also in Daoist inner alchemy to refine *jing* back into *qi*. Moving *qi* along the Conception and Governing Vessels, practitioners activate various uniquely Daoist points, such as the cinnabar fields in the head, chest, and abdomen; the Three Passes, located at the coccyx (GV-1), the heart (GV-10), and the occiput (GV-17); and the third eye, an extra point on the Governing Vessel known as Hall of Yin (Yintang) or Spirit Pass (Shenguan), the entrance to the Nine Palaces in the head.

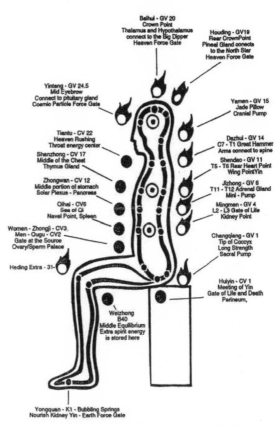

Fig. 10. The microcosmic orbit.

There is a certain similarity of the Daoist use of the vessels with the Indian practice of Kundalini Yoga. In Ayurvedic medicine and the yogic tradition, the body is vitalized by a set of seven energy centers or chakras, located along the spine. They, too, begin at the pelvic floor, with the Root Chakra at the perineum, then move up through the Sacral Chakra at the level of the abdomen and the Central Chakra at the solar plexus to the Heart Chakra in the chest. From here three further centers are the Throat Chakra at the top of the spine, the Brow Chakra, also known as the Third Eye, and finally the Crown Chakra at the top of the head.

The belief is that life's universal energy, known as *shakti*, manifests in the body in a hidden but highly potent form, called *kundalini*. Similar to a serpent, this force lies curled at the bottom of the spine, to be awakened by spiritual practices or the touch of a guru. Once activated, the serpent uncoils and moves slowly through the chakras to the top of the head, where it joins with cosmic *shakti* and opens the individual to a celestial connection and the attainment of transcendence and liberation. The Daoist vision is rather similar in that here, too, energy flows up the spine, is refined into purer forms, and eventually aids the practitioner in attaining access to otherworldly dimensions and the joys of immortality. The main difference is that while in Indian practice the *kundalini* moves in a linear motion to connect with *brahman* above, in Daoism the movement is circular, going both up and down to effect a thorough refinement of *qi* before allowing it to exit the body through the top of the head and to communicate with the gods. Chinese medical practice, by harmonizing the *qi*-flow in the twelve major meridians, creates the preconditions of health necessary for the successful pursuit of the higher spiritual goals.

Further Readings

Ellis, Andrew, Nigel Wiseman, and Ken Boss. 1989. *Grasping the Wind: An Exploration into the Meaning of the Chinese Acupuncture Point Names*. Brookline, Mass.: Paradigm Publications.

Kaptchuk, Ted J. 1983. *The Web that Has No Weaver: Understanding Chinese Medicine*. New York: Congdon & Weed.

Kendall, Donald E. 2002. *Dao of Chinese Medicine: Understanding an Ancient Healing Art*. New York: Oxford University Press.

Larre, Claude, and Elisabeth Rochat de la Vallee. 1996. *Eight Extraordinary Vessels*. Cambridge: Monkey Press.

Maciocia, Giovanni. 1989. *The Foundations of Chinese Medicine: A Comprehensive Text for Acupuncturists and Herbalists*. New York: Churchill Livingstone.

Matsumoto, Kiiko, and Stephen Birch. 1986. *Extraordinary Vessels*. Brookline, Mass.: Paradigm Books.

Reid, David P. 2000. *The Complete Guide to Chi-Gung*. Boston: Shambhala.

Seem, Mark D. 1990. *Acupuncture Imaging: Perceiving the Energy Pathways of the Body*. New York: Inner Traditions.

Willmont, Dennis. 2001. *The Twelve Spirit Points of Acupuncture*. Marchfield, Mass.: Willmountain Press.

Chapter 6
Methods of Diagnosis

To find out where a given person stands in the process of healing and self-realization, various methods of diagnosis are applied in the Chinese health system. Diagnosis means the process of taking in data on the patient's health situation and evaluating them in terms of yin and yang, excess and deficiency, while finding the specific location of energetic imbalance. It involves a broad application of correlative thinking, taking all the different aspects of a patient's life into account.

The word for "symptom" in Chinese is *zheng*. It indicates the concrete manifestation of an imbalance on three different levels. First, it denotes the initial "signs" of an illness, which may still be very subtle and perceived merely as a slight irregularity by the patient. Second, it indicates the specific "symptoms" of the disease, detected by the physician in a thorough examination. And third, it means the "syndrome" constituting the illness, revealing the larger pattern of disharmony both in the body and the social life of the patient.

The goal of Chinese medical diagnostics is syndrome differentiation, i.e., to find an underlying pattern of disharmony and identify the main organ and meridian gone astray. This stands in contrast to Western medicine, which usually looks for one single point where the illness starts. Chinese diagnosis accordingly examines many different dimensions of the person and includes all symptoms present, such as physical pains, emotions, social situations, environmental factors, and so on.

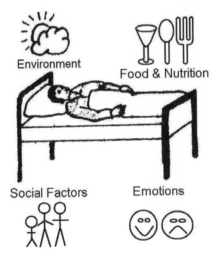

Fig. 11. The patient in context.

63

The worldview behind this understanding has been described as "synchronicity," the consideration of different aspects of life coinciding at one single moment in time as opposed to the examination of the same area or symptom over a longer period. In Western culture, synchronicity is used for example in astrology where the movements of the planets are related to human fate and emotions. As a serious way of looking at the world it was described by the psychologist C. G. Jung who defined it as a bridge between the outer world and inner reality, an apparently causeless order in the present moment, the overlapping of subjective and objective realities. His most prominent example is the story of an interview with a patient who was telling him a dream about a scarab while a very similar looking beetle appeared on the window sill. Other synchronous events are the ringing of the telephone just as we are thinking of someone we have not heard from in years; the continued appearance of certain numbers that for some reason have caught our attention; and the apparently unrelated presence of certain symptoms and certain states of mind (Jung, *Interpretations*). The understanding of the world as a synchronous network in addition to linear causality is central to Chinese medical thinking and plays an important role in diagnosis.

In concrete practice, diagnosis begins with data collection through four inspections or examinations: looking, asking, listening/smelling, and touching. Looking consists of observing the patient from the most outer to the most inner components. The patient inevitably comes with some complaint, but before addressing it the practitioner looks at who the patient is (see www.internalhealers.com). The first level of inspection is at the level of *shen* or spirit. If the patient is lively, well animated and with rosy cheeks, makes eye contact, and generally seems healthy, the prognosis for recovery is good. In this case the patient is said to have good *shen* or spirit. If the patient is slow, dull in response, heavy in body motion, and generally ill at ease, the prognosis is more difficult, and the patient is considered to have poor or lacking *shen*. This principle holds true for all visual inspections.

> **Exercise:** Look through magazines and find three pictures of people who look healthy and exude good *shen*. Then find three pictures of people who look sickly and are examples of poor *shen*. Share them with your classmates. Also, observe people walking in the street: are they happy, outgoing, walking upright with clear eyes; or are they depressed, withdrawing, and hunched forward?

The presence or lack of *shen* reveals the fundamental aspect of yin and yang as seen in visual diagnosis and indicates the state of the body's recovery ability. The term *shen* or spirit is employed since it is considered the most yang of the body's core substances. As such, it is considered to emanate from the body and produce the overall impressions that each of us perceives even on some subtle level.

Beyond the examination of *shen*, visual diagnosis examines the colors associated with the internal organs on the surface of the skin: liver—green, heart—red, spleen—yellow, lungs—white, and kidneys—black. Natural and resonant manifestations of the organs, these colors appear in near equal emission when the person is healthy. In an imbalanced state, which may not yet show true pathological symptoms, the balance of colors will be off, more severely so for more serious conditions.

For the sensitive practitioner, the color imbalance can be perceived as emanating from the body, almost like an aura—described in the West as a single or multiple-hued layer of energy surrounding the body that reflects the person's inherent nature and that can be photographed with the help of Kirlian photography (see www.kirlian.org). Most commonly, however, Chinese practitioners look for specific places to identify the quality of colors, such as the sclera of the eyes, the skin under the eyes, the temples, the skin by the nose, the lips, and the forearms.

Exercise: Look at the people in your environment and try to find someone who evidences each of the five phase colors. Ask them about their health. Do the colors match their health concerns?

In addition to color diagnosis, the body type is visually inspected. Each of the phases is associated with a type of tissue, and a person with an abundance of such tissue is considered to be of the corresponding phase constitution. Wood is associated with joints and tendons, fire with blood vessels, earth with muscle, metal with skin, and water with bone. If the patient is wiry and has visible sinews, the odds are that he is a wood body type. If the patient is fleshy and round, she may be an earth body type. This part of visual diagnosis is also influenced by the patient's individual history and habits, since poor diet and lack of exercise make every body type overweight. However, it is used mainly to determine the patient's general tendencies and to provide a backdrop for the understanding of the evolution of a pathology.

Perhaps the most central component of visual inspection is the tongue. The tongue is considered a mirror of the body: its tip matches the head and its root the pelvis, and its different sections correspond to the organs. Examining the tongue allows the practitioner to inspect the state of the body's internal balance.

He or she begins by observing the presence or absence of *shen*. Just like in the body in general, a lively, well shaped tongue has good *shen* and indicates a good prognosis. Once the *shen* is observed, then the tongue is inspected for its coating, shape, and color.

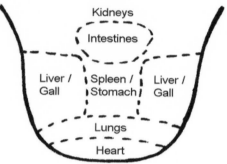

Fig. 12. The Inner Organs on the Tongue.

The coating or "moss" of the tongue indicates the relative state of body fluids in a continuum from no coat through thick coat to peeled coat, with multiple variations in between. The absence of a coat may indicate a lack of the stomach fluids necessary to generate a coat. The thickness of a coat indicates the relative thickness of the body fluids. A thin white coat is considered normal and indicative of a relative fluid balance. If the coat is very thin and clear, the fluids are deficient and the body lacks the ability to lubricate its membranes and joints.

If the coat is thick, the fluids are sluggish and the patient may have internal cold, which congests fluids as if freezing them, or dampness which is the accumulation of turbid body fluids. If the fluid congestion continues for a long time, the tongue coat will look greasy and be indicative of a state known as phlegm, which implies a stopping of the fluid flow often leading to masses, growths, and tumors. The coat may also peel off the tongue, leaving a shiny surface. This peeled look reveals a more severe imbalance, often typified by the correspondence of the peeled spot to an area of the body. Then again, the tongue coat may have a coloring. A white coat often relates to cold; a yellow coat, to heat. In extreme cases, the coat can even become black which indicates a potentially fatal cold invasion.

The shape of the tongue is evaluated for whether it is short or long, swollen or thin, cracked or smooth, and for the presence or absence of visible veins. A swollen tongue seems too large for the mouth. Often the sides of the tongue appear wavy in a pattern known as "teeth marks" or "scalloping." This is caused by the swelling between the ligaments which hold the tongue together and cause it to flare out at its lateral edges. Mechanically the swollen tongue is indicative of a relative imbalance between interstitial fluid and blood fluid volumes; essentially the tissues are water logged. The swollen tongue is clinically related to weak spleen yang which is responsible for transformation of the fluids. This presentation often also evidences edema in the joints as well as a puffy appearance. When the tongue is thin, it indicates a deficiency in the blood which should fill the tongue. This is considered a precursor to yin deficiency, evidenced by dry signs on the mucus membrane as well as insomnia, irritability, hot flashes, and amenorrhea.

Cracks in the tongue indicate a long-standing disharmony of the organs matching specific areas of the tongue. Finally, the underside of the tongue is inspected for the visibility of veins. If the veins are dark and visible, the overall circulatory system is inefficient—like the hands of an arthritic patient who develops darker veins due to the poor circulation. The color of the body of the tongue is the last parameter inspected. If the tongue is pale and washed out, the *qi* is deficient. If the tongue is dark, black, or purple, the blood is stagnant. These colors can be general to the tongue body or they can be local to a given correspondence area.

> **Exercise:** Go to www.yinyanghouse.com or to io.uwinnipeg.ca/~hali/doc/tonguediagnosis/td.html and diagnose several different tongues on the basis of their major characteristics. Then try your skills on a friend or two. For a self-diagnosis, see www.beyondwellbeing.com.

The next part of diagnosis is asking. Specific questions based on the functions of the organs are asked to tease out the functioning of the inner aspects of the body. The ten traditional areas of inquiry include: appetite, digestion, elimination, activity, sweat, sleep, menstruation, sexual health, reproduction, and demeanor (see www.chinesemedicinesampler.com; www.internalhealers.com). Inquiring about specific symptoms as well as about diet, sexual activity, exercise, social relationships, and overall likes and dislikes, the practitioner will analyze the patient's answers and note certain data. For example, too much raw food can cause dampness, while lots of hot, greasy food can create internal heat; too much exercise causes the *qi* to flow too fast and enhances excess in the organs, while lack of exercise can create deficiencies. She may also look for typical patterns, such as kidney deficiency, common in the West, which manifests in lower back pain, frequent urination, knee pain, low energy levels, black circles under the eyes, joint discomfort, low sex drive, and anxiety. It usually relates to a life-style that involves sexual overindulgence, too much caffeine, pollution, or stress which may appear in any area of the patient's life. All this is flushed out in asking diagnosis.

Next come listening and smelling: the most unobtrusive inspections. They are grouped together because in classical Chinese the word *wen* means both "to hear" and "to smell," expressing a sensory connection the Chinese perceived between these two activities. Usually the patient may not even know she is being inspected in this way. The physician listens carefully to her sound of voice, the quality of her speech, even the decisiveness or hesitancy in dealing with an authority figure. Listening may even happen over the phone, providing a first impression of the patient and giving clues to some underlying energetic patterns. Similarly smelling is done very subtly, the healer taking in the body odor and quality of breath of the person and classifying it in terms of the five phases, thus gaining an initial sense of what imbalance there might be.

Listening diagnosis uses the five-phases system to typify the patient's voice and determine either the underlying constitutional tendency or the most imbalanced phase. Wood relates to shouting, fire to laughing, earth to singing, metal to weeping, and water to groaning. If the patient's voice can be associated with one of these sounds, the related phase is suspect.

The last of the four inspections, touching diagnosis, is perhaps the most central of the traditional diagnostic system. The meridians and points are touched, the abdomen is palpated, and the pulse is taken. Touching these areas provides a plethora of information for the practitioner. First, any symptomatic area is touched. This means that an aching shoulder is palpated for range of motion and pain. Touching also inspects the relative *qi*-flow through the meridians which traverse the area, as well as the points which may have special influence over it. Presence or absence of pain and levels of heat or cold are noted. Tautness may indicate excess; slackness may be a sign of deficiency. Often long-standing problems manifest as numbness in the relevant treatment points, which is a sign of poor prognosis. The abdomen is palpated as an indicator of both five phases and meridian patterns of disharmony.

Finally, the pulse is taken as a major index of the body's state. The pulse most commonly used is the radial pulse, although the carotid and mallear pulses are traditionally employed as well. The radial pulse is subdivided into three divisions from the wrist crease upward along the arm and parted into three depths. This creates eighteen positions that are cross-referenced to twenty-eight possible quality assessments, eventually resulting in a diagnostic pattern. Due to its complexity, it takes decades to become skilled at pulse diagnosis. The pulse is always taken in three positions and on both sides, and by applying three different pressures — superficial, medium, and deep — each matching the quality of *qi* in two of the twelve key organs (see www.americanacupuncture.com):

1. left: heart/small intestine   1. right: lungs/large intestine
2. left: liver/gall bladder   2. right: spleen/stomach
3. left: kidney/bladder   3. right: pericardium/triple heater

The twenty-eight types of pulses, then, consist of eighteen classes distinguished according to depth (2), speed (2), width (2), strength (2), shape (4), length (2), rhythm (3), and balance (1); plus ten types, i.e., flooding, minute, frail, soggy, leathery, hidden, confined, spinning, hollow, and scattered. The most desirable pulse is moderate, regular, medium, strong, and even (see www.yinyanghouse.com). When taking the patient's pulse, variants due to seasons, time of day, and gender must be taken into consideration. All other abnormalities indicate weakness or excess of the *qi* in specific organs. Typical indications include:

Type	Feeling	Indication
superficial	easily palpable but weak	beginning disease
deep	felt only with pressure	internal syndromes
slow	less than four beats	cold syndromes
rapid	more than five beats	heat syndromes
taut	forceful and tight	yang hyperactivity
wry	rolling or flowing	excessive phlegm
thready	rather fine pulse	deficient *qi*/blood
short	uneven, missing beats	*qi*/blood-stagnation
knotted	slow, irregular misses	endogenous cold
intermittent	slow, regular misses	impairment of *qi*

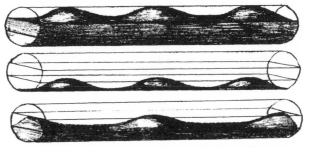

Fig. 13. The superficial, deep, and slow pulses.

> **Exercise:** Feel someone's pulse in the positions described and try to classify it in accordance with the various types. What is a likely diagnosis?

After gathering data from the four inspections, the practitioner tries to come to a coherent understanding to account for the current state of affairs. The etiology and pathology of the case culminate in a pattern of the balance of the body's energies, fluids, and structure and ideally provide the course of treatment. To find this, two steps are taken. First, information is classified in terms of the six pernicious influences and eight principal patterns; second, the information is linked with one or two dominant organs and meridians to be addressed in treatment.

The six pernicious influences are the classical origins of disease in Chinese thinking. The eight principal patterns are four pairs of yin-yang based opposites that describe systematic symptoms. Both appear first in medical literature in *On Cold-Induced Disorders* (*Shanghan lun*) of the third century C.E., a text that reflects an herbal-based alternative to the five phases system and was later integrated into the dominant model.

The six pernicious influences are classified into yin and yang and each are divided into two aspects: external (those that invade the body) and internal (those generated in the body).

The three yang influences are:

1. Wind, i.e., fast change or movement in the body, associated with the liver. Manifests first on the body surface, may appear as pain, skin eruptions, fever, and fear of drafts. It can also be an internally generated, chronic liver problem.

2. Heat, i.e., acceleration or dilation, linked with the heart. Symptoms include red skin, swellings, inflammation, yellow secretions, dry tongue, thirst, rapid pulse, perspiration, red face, fever, and swollen throat. The patient appears agitated and talkative, thirsty, and constipated.

3. Dryness, i.e., withering or shriveling tendency, related to the lungs. Manifests as asthma, phlegm, fever, body aches, dry nostrils, tongue, or skin, and lack of urination. It indicates an internal loss of fluids and often comes with irritation, weakness, or anemia.

The three yin influences are:

4. Cold, i.e., contraction or retardation, linked with the kidneys. Patient appears pale, cold, contracted, with clear se-

cretions. He may have a fever but no sweat, and tends to feel cold, stiff, or sleepy; appears shrinking and clenching, is quiet and unwilling to talk, shows a lack of thirst, and tends toward diarrhea.

5. Dampness, i.e., sinking or accumulating, related to the spleen. Generates turbid, sticky, or cloudy secretions, feelings of nausea, swellings, a greasy tongue, as well as heavy or sore limbs. Patients often have oily skin and indigestion.

6. Summer heat, i.e., drying out, linked with the pericardium. Caused by exposure to extreme heat, it creates exhaustion, depletion of fluids, sweating, and bursts of high fever.

Usually the picture presented by the patient is a mixture of these various general indications, from which a dominant pattern is identified. For example, the presence of an obstruction of *qi* could be caused by cold or by heat. If it is cold-induced, there will be a pale skin and complexion, a white coat on the tongue, and a dislike of cold. Such an obstruction tends to be long-term or chronic; it comes from an insufficient flow of *qi* to the area in question. A heat-induced obstruction, on the other hand, shows an overflow of *qi* that is moving fast in different directions and thus creates blockages. This is a more acute obstruction. The patient will show redness and swelling, and express a strong liking for coolness and cold substances. The treatment various accordingly: cooling herbs and drainage for the heat-induced disorder; warming compresses, teas, and medicines, as well as enhancement of *qi* through acupuncture for the cold one.

Cold and heat are also a pair in the eight principal patterns, together with interior and exterior, deficiency and excess, and yin and yang. The goal in this part of the diagnostic process is to get a sense of the fundamental yin or yang nature of the disease. Yin qualities include *cold* symptoms as described above; *interior* symptoms, i.e., chronic conditions, digestive problems including vomiting, loose stool, and a sinking puls; and signs of *deficiency*, such as frail, weak movements, a low voice, pale face and tongue, shallow breath, pain relieved by pressure, copious urination, and a weak pulse. Yang symptoms are at the opposite end of the spectrum, including *heat*-induced phenomena; *exterior* symptoms, i.e., an acute illness with aversion to cold and wind, fever, body aches, and a floating pulse; and signs of *qi* in *excess*, such as ponderous and forceful movements, a loud voice, thick tongue moss, heavy breathing, pain aggravated by pressure, and a full and heavy pulse.

It is natural to have a patient whose symptoms and responses fall into more than one of these categories, but it is the task of the analytical practitioner to discern a dominant energetic pattern that will fit the overall condition into a more yin or a more yang basic pattern. If done by systematic check list, all the various data taken through the four inspections would be listed in a complex chart divided according to yin and yang, and the area with the most checks would form the basis of diagnosis. More commonly, the practitioner relies on experience and personal impressions rather than the mechanical counting of symptoms. He or she is alert for telltale signs and, as the patient explains the complaint and undergoes examination, classifies key characteristics into *qi*-flow patterns.

Once a baseline of yin and yang has been established, the one remaining question is where the imbalance is located among the meridians so that treatment can begin. For the most part, this is fairly obvious from the symptoms presented. For example, lack of appetite, abdominal pain that is relieved by touch, and loose stool are indicative of a deficiency in the stomach area and can initially be approached through the spleen and stomach meridians. The problem may be solved here, or treatment may lead to the arising of different symptoms, showing an underlying imbalance in another organ and meridian. Similarly, in a case of cold, caught when unprotected in cold weather, with stuffy nose, slight fever, hardship in breathing, and body aches, the most likely meridian to be affected is the lung. Since the yin organs are considered the storage centers of *qi*, most diagnoses will come down to a description in their terms, e.g., Deficient Spleen *Qi*, Cold Violating the Lungs, or Rising Liver Fire (Kaptchuk, *Web*, ch. 8).

The Chinese understand diseases in terms of the increased invasion and malfunctioning of different layers of the body's energetic system. The first level, harming energies toward the outside of the body, involve problems with defensive or protective *qi* and manifest in frequent colds or allergies. Second is *qi*, whose disturbance may lead to chronic sinus infections, asthma, skin disorders, and persistent digestive problems, such as irritable bowel syndrome. Third, and further toward the body's interior, is blood. When harmed, it will lead to yet more serious conditions, including arthritis, lupus, diabetes, and chronic fatigue syndrome. Fourth and finally, when the inner organs themselves are impacted, major and often terminal diseases result, such as AIDS and the various forms of cancer (Elias, *Five Elements of Self-Healing*). It is thus important that conditions are recognized and corrected early, so that disturbances never reach the deeper levels. The further advanced a disease, the harder it is to correct and the more changes will have to be made in lifestyle and identity of the patient.

Three major levels of treatment complexity can accordingly be distinguished. The most straightforward level involves ailments that are acute, exterior caused, and immediately treatable, such as a cold caught in freezing weather, a headache due to exposure to the sun or noxious fumes, an injury of an arm or leg, or a stomach upset due to bad food. The symptoms are clearly localized, the origin of the condition is fairly obvious, and treatment is undertaken while the situation is still fresh. Prognosis in these cases is excellent, since the pattern is clear and the symptoms are recent.

A second level of treatment is somewhat more complex. The symptoms may be clearly localized but the behavioral examination and the pulses indicate the presence of wayward *qi* also in other areas. The disease is not presented for treatment when first indications arise, but the patient has lived with it for some time, allowing its imbalance to spread into different areas of the body. An injury of the right leg, for example, that was thought to have healed may have caused a heavier burden on the left leg which in turn affected the hips, spine, and shoulders. The patient complains of back pain, but the ultimate cause has little to do with the back.

Or there may be a person with persistent headaches, apparently related to neck tension but in fact the result of dietary habits and a spleen or liver imbalance. In these cases, the clinician will take into account the multiple layers of the pattern and begin treatment with the most dominant meridian affected, which may or may not be the one indicated by the obvious symptoms. A sequence of treatments will gradually clear up the dominant pattern and allow the underlying symptoms to come forth.

The third level of treatment is the most complex. It is necessitated in cases of deep-seated or chronic disorders that the patient has lived with for years and that have impacted not only on one or two meridians but have come to shape his or her identity and ways of acting in the world — physically, emotionally, dietetically, even socially. The wider intake of information on lifestyle, family, work, and the person's overall situation is very important here. Patterns appear that seem to be revolving spirals of symptoms and indications, beginning with an obvious surface one that can be addressed immediately, but whose resolution will only bring out deeper levels of imbalance that cause more discomfort. Prognosis varies widely in these complex situations, since patients tend to be attached to their conditions and lifestyles and often are reluctant to change who they are in order to become healthy. Questions of identity, self-image, and spiritual quest arise here, and the physician moves out of the realm of strict healing and into the area of personal and cosmic growth.

Further Readings

Aziz, Robert. 1990. *C. G. Jung's Psychology of Religion and Synchronicity*. Albany: State University of New York Press.

Beinfeld, Harriet, and Efram Kormbold. 1991. *Between Heaven and Earth: A Guide to Chinese Medicine*. New York: Ballentine Books.

Elias, Jason, and Katherine Ketcham. 1998. *The Five Elements of Self-Healing: Using Chinese Medicine for Maximum Immunity, Wellness, and Health*. New York: Harmony Books.

Jung, C. G. 1955. *The Interpretation of Nature and the Psyche: Synchronicity*. London: Routledge & Kegan Paul.

Kaptchuk, Ted J. 1983. *The Web that Has No Weaver: Understanding Chinese Medicine*. New York: Congdon & Weed.

Krippner, Stanley, and Daniel Rubin, eds. 1974. *Galaxies of Life: A Conference on Kirlian Photography, Acupuncture, and the Human Aura*. Garden City, N.J.: Anchor Books.

Liu, Yanzhi. 1988. *The Essential Book of Traditional Chinese Medicine*. 2 Vols. New York: Columbia University Press.

Mitchell, Craig, Feng Ye, and Nigel Wiseman. 1999. *Shang Han Lun: On Cold Damage*. Brookline, Mass.: Paradigm Publications.

Peat, F. David. 1992. *Synchronicity: The Bridge Between Matter and Mind*. New York, Bantam Books.

Porkert, Manfred. 1983. *The Essentials of Chinese Diagnosis*. Zürich: Acta Medicinae Sinensis.

Chapter 7
Acupuncture

Acupuncture, a seventeenth-century term based on the Latin word *acus* (needle), is called *zhenjiu* in Chinese, literally "needles and moxa." It means the insertion of fine needles into specific points along the meridians to regulate the flow of *qi* through tonification or dispersal. "To tonify means to strengthen the normal *qi* so that diminished function is restored. Dispersal means to promote the expulsion of pathogenic influences or excess, again to restore normal body function" (Chen and Wang, *Acupuncture Case Histories*, 11). In addition, acupuncture commonly also involves moxibustion, i.e., the burning of moxa (mugwort, *artemisia vulgaris*) on relevant acupuncture points to enhance the effect of the treatment, and a follow-up treatment with herbs.

Historically acupuncture appears first in Han-dynasty sources, i.e., texts from the beginning of the Common Era. Its origins are unclear. One argument says that it was discovered when soldiers were wounded by arrows in battle and upon recovery found that their various other diseases had disappeared together with the injury. Another argument, presented by Paul Unschuld in *Medicine in China*, speaks of demon medicine based on a form primitive thinking that saw the cause of sickness outside the body and located it predominantly in the supernatural realm. Thus the earliest Chinese character for "sickness" (*ji*) shows the combined picture of a bed and an arrow, signifying that the person was hit by a supernatural arrow and is now lying prone on his bed. The character for "doctor" (*yi*) consists of an arrow in a box together with a lance and a pitcher of wine, revealing the military-style repertory of early physicians. Also, many medical texts speak of disease "invading" while physicians "attack" and "vanquish" it.

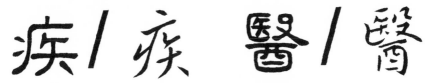

Fig. 14. The Chinese characters for "sickness" and "physician."

Another speculation on the origins of acupuncture maintains that it developed from the treatment of boils and abscesses with pointed stones in conjunction with the practice of bloodletting to release wayward *qi*. This practice, joined by an elementary connection of extremities to inner organs, is also known from ancient Greece and may indicate a possible contact among the ancient cultures (see Kuriyama, *Expressiveness*). It is also documented that cramps, numbness, and paralysis were treated with needles in south China from an early period. As part of this theory, scholars suggest that the burning of moxa preceded acupuncture and that the needles were later added to support and help it. This is supported by evidence from the Mawangdui manuscripts.

In 1973, fifteen medical manuscripts written on silk, bamboo, and strips of wood, were excavated from tomb no. 3 at Mawangdui near Changsha (Hunan). Dated to 168 B.C.E., they include several important early texts on ways to harmonize yin and yang, find alignment with the Dao, nourish life through herbs, breathing exercises, sexual techniques, as well as methods of absorbing *qi*, abstaining from grains, and undertaking therapeutic gymnastics (Harper, *Early Chinese Medical Manuscripts*). The texts describe various healing modalities, including moxibustion, spells, rituals, gymnastics, sexual practices, drugs, massages, cupping, bathing, and fumigation, but no acupuncture. Needles are mentioned only as a means to open abscesses in the body and to apply pressure to hemorrhoids. The main method used to stimulate *qi* in the body is moxibustion (see Engelhardt, "Neue Funde").

More specifically, the texts know of eleven meridians, associated with the five yin and six yang organs. However, they do not call them meridians (*jingluo*) but arteries or vessels (*mai*), thus expressing a concept of *qi* linked intimately with the blood and its circulation. It was only in the first major medical text, the *Yellow Emperor's Inner Classic*, a collection of texts from several medical schools of the Han dynasty, that a twelfth meridian was added for symmetry. Also in this text the blood vessels were first separated from the meridian system, thus establishing two different networks of circulation in the body. The concept of *qi* became more abstract and was classified as a major yang vitality, while the blood was seen in more cosmic and energetic terms as a key yin vitality, although it never lost its concrete meaning (see www.acupuncturecare.com; www.drfreely. com/acupuncture/history).

The *Yellow Emperor's Inner Classic* is the single most important text of Chinese medicine. It consists of a dialogue between the Yellow Emperor

(Huangdi) and various medical masters who teach him how to understand and heal the human body. It describes how the Dao underlies all as universal harmony, how yin and yang establish the world, and how the body is organized and works. Relying on phase energetics, it outlines the major methods of diagnosis and key types of diseases, recommending not only immediate cures but also long-term adjustments in lifestyle through calming the spirit, regulating the diet, and taking proper exercise. It deals extensively with the practice of acupuncture.

The *Yellow Emperor's Inner Classic* consists of four separate texts, which in contents go back to the Han dynasty but were edited later. The most important is the *Yellow Emperor's Simple Questions* (*Huangdi neijing suwen*; trl. Veith 1972; Lu 1987; Ni 1995), where the Yellow Emperor is in dialogue with the mythical physician Qi Bo. Its surviving edition was compiled by Wang Bing and dates from 762. A second version is the *Yellow Emperor's Divine Pivot* (*Huangdi neijing lingshu*; trl. Ki 1985; Wu 1993), edited by Yang Shanshan around the year 600. It contains similar materials as the *Simple Questions* but presents different partners of the Yellow Emperor and is an indication of different schools within acupuncture.

A third text of the same group is the *Yellow Emperor's Classic of Great Simplicity* (*Huangdi neijing taisu*), also edited around the year 600 but not translated to date. The fourth and last work is the *Yellow Emperor's Classic of 81 Difficult Issues* (*Huangdi bashiyi nanjing*; trl. Unschuld 1986), which was transmitted as a key manual to Korea and Japan and has remained popular among acupuncturists there. It is divided into eighty-one parts that each begin with a question or "difficult issue," which is then addressed in detail. This text, too, is in dialogue format and presents essentially the same material as the *Simple Questions*, but it is more integrated, better organized, and reveals a more complex system of different schools, pathologies, and diagnoses joined together. All three texts received numerous commentaries and were reorganized variously by medical masters.

A comprehensive summary of much of the same material was created in 282 C.E. by Huangfu Mi and is known as the *Systematic Classic of Acupuncture and Moxibustion* (*Zhenjiu jiayi jing*). "The oldest extant technical book devoted to acupuncture and moxibustion" (Lu, *Celestial Lancets*, 122), this already lists 649 of the 670 acupuncture points commonly used today. It is the first extant text to emphasize acupuncture as a means of disease prevention, providing detailed descriptions of the meridians, point names and locations, as well as needling techniques. From the same period stems also the *Pulse Classic* (*Maijing*) by Wang Shuhe (210-286 C.E.) which describes twenty-four pulses with analytical diagnoses. The book served to establish the study of pulses as an independent branch of Chinese medicine.

Exercise: Get a copy of one of the classical texts in translation and read two or three chapters. What strikes you most about the discourse? How is medical knowledge transmitted in these works?

These and other classics (*jing*) constituted the highest type of medical literature in traditional China. They discussed overarching questions and defined a canonical level of information. Next came a group of texts called discussions (*lun*), which were devoted to the theoretical understanding of specific pathological states or causes. A third class of medical literature was called prescriptions (*fang*). It encompassed treatment records, notes, anecdotes, and personal insights with little theoretical explanation. Beyond written medical works, many techniques and recipes were also transmitted orally from master to disciple, thus enlivening the tradition and creating the multifaceted medical system of today.

One aid to memorization of acupuncture channels and points has been the use of human figurines, first discovered in a wooden statue with meridian lines and point markings that was unearthed in Sichuan in southwest China and dates from the second century B.C.E. Similarly, a bronze figurine from the eleventh century shows remnants of mercury and wax at indentations marking points. Written documents explain that these indentations were filled with mercury and covered with wax for examination purposes. When a candidate at a prefectural or imperial medical school correctly stabbed the point, the mercury would flow out, and he would pass the exam. Similar statues are still common today, mostly made from plastic and painted with lines in different colors.

Acupuncturists in traditional China used needles made from various materials. The earliest needles from stone, thorns, bamboo, or bone, were later replaced by metal — iron, copper, bronze, gold, and silver. Steel was not discovered until the middle of the fifth century C.E. and only sufficiently developed for acupuncture practice around the year 800. Still "acupuncture could never have reached the height of its effectiveness, administering its stimuli while causing the minimum of injury to the tissues, without wire-thin, and therefore metallic, needles" (Lu, *Celestial Lancets*, 73). The stainless steel, disposable needle is still standard today.

The needles, moreover, came in various forms, many of which are still in use today. Most common are thin needles of medium length used for general acupuncture. Sharp arrowheads are used for superficial or shal-low needling, applied to par-ticularly sore areas, as well as in children and the elderly. Nee-dles with a soft, rounded top are used for local massage. Those with a blunt head help to exert pressure in specific areas. Three-edged needles are used to punc-ture veins; sword-like needles help to drain abscesses; sharp and round ones are for rapid pricking; and very long needles, up to five or six inches, are used for joints and solid tissue areas. Contemporary Chinese needles tend to be longer and thicker than those used in Korea and Ja-pan, where they are as thin as a hair and come in a plastic tube for keeping and easy insertion.

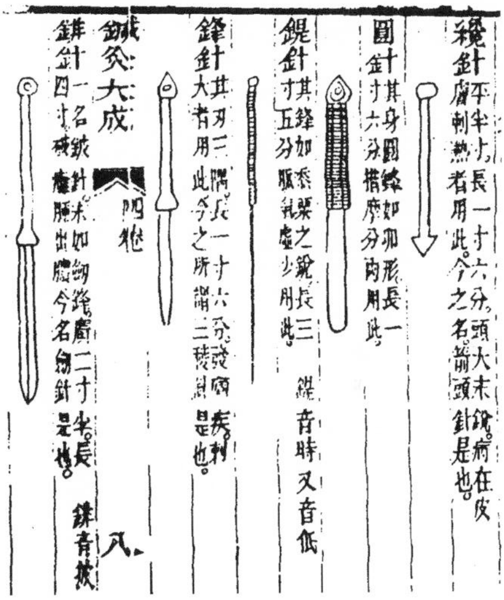

Fig. 15. Types and shapes of acupuncture needles.

Before inserting a needle, the practitioner finds the correct point by exert-ing pressure in the area where it should be located. The point is found when the spot is sensitive and slightly sore to the touch, or the skin forms a slight hollow or a distinct mound. Then he or she inserts the needle, holding it between the thumb and index finger of one hand while tightening the skin with the other. The most common angle of insertion is 90 degrees, but on the chest, head, and arms it is often also 45 degrees, usually in the direction of *qi*-flow, or even only 15-25 degrees in more sensitive areas, such as the top of head or near the eyes.

To enhance the *qi*-giving power, the needle can be raised and lowered or twirled and rotated a few times after insertion, using movements that often have exotic names, like "circling dragon," "fire on the mountain," or "three emanations of heaven." Balanced raising and lowering ensures that the meridian is both tonified and drained equally. A deeper, slower lowering causes tonification, while a more shallow, faster lowering cre-ates drainage. Similarly, small twirling and rotation ensures tonification, while larger, more extensive rotation causes the *qi* to drain. Also, the needle can be placed in the direction of the meridian to enhance tonification or against it to provide draining. Should a stronger effect be desired, the skin may also be pressed outward from the needle and along the meridian to encourage *qi*-flow.

> **Exercise:** Go back to the points in chapter 5. Find some on your body and press on them with your thumb or forefinger. Are any of them sore? Do the areas show up as mounds or hollows? Do you have any symptoms associated with them? Massage a few of them, pushing in different directions and with varying intensity. Can you feel *qi* moving?

To protect himself or herself, the practitioner should synchronize breathing with that of the patient and ideally insert needles on a mutual exhalation. This prevents large amounts of wayward *qi* flowing directly into the practitioner. There should be neither blood nor pain when a needle is inserted, although certain spots can be sensitive. However, there should be a definite feeling of "getting *qi*" (*deqi*). This can be felt both at the insertion point and in the area of symptoms. For the patient, getting *qi* means a sense of warmth and vitality when a point is tonified, and a sense of coolness, release, or opening when *qi* is drained. The practitioner, too, can feel the arrival of *qi*, sensing a fullness and stronger pulse in cases of successful tonification, and receiving a feeling of tension and contraction under the needle and a lesser pulse in cases of drainage. The rule of thumb is that the faster *deqi* is achieved, the better the prognosis.

Once the *qi* has arrived, the needles may be taken out again immediately or left in place for ten or more minutes to keep up stimulation. In some complex cases, and as guided by some practitioners, needles are left in even longer, for half an hour or more. The time of continued stimulation allows the patient's system to adjust to the new balance created in the body, activating his or her own innate healing powers and homeostatic functions. The same process is repeated twice, once for the front and once for the back of the body.

Other acupuncture techniques include cutaneous needling, where a delicate hammer-head instrument called a plum blossom needle is tapped lightly over the skin in the direction of meridian flow (in cases of severe deficiency); bloodletting, where a sharp, triangular needle is inserted in a specific point to release some blood (in cases of excess heat or high fever); piercing, where the skin is pierced open and underlying fibers are severed with a large needle or knife (in cases of skin eruptions); and cupping, where a vacuum is created in a round glass vial by passing an open flame inside it, then the vial is quickly placed on the skin where it pulls the flesh and muscles upward, thus stimulating an entire area.

Supplementing the needles is the practice of moxibustion, the burning of mugwort or artemisia on the body. Collected best in the fifth month, the herb is thoroughly dried in the sun, then ground into a powdery substance. It is applied in four ways: moxa cones, moxa cigars, moxa boxes, and moxa on needles. The most common are moxa cones. Small amounts of the powdered herb are shaped into small cones, which are then dried again in the sun so that the oils evaporate and the herb burns slowly. The cone is placed either directly on the skin or on top of a small buffer, such as a layer of salt or a slice of fresh ginger or garlic. With a lighted incense stick, the cone is set afire and burns slowly down. If placed directly on the skin, it can either be extinguished as soon as the heat reaches the body or be allowed to burn down to leave a scar. The latter is used mainly for chronic conditions in patients with a strong constitution. Usually moxa is applied several times to the same point.

Moxa cigars are long, rolled up cylinders that contain larger portions of the herb. They are lighted at the front and held about one inch above the chosen point to create a sense of heat and *qi*-flow. They may be removed at times by raising the cigar, then lowered again, over a period of several minutes. The moxa box is a small wooden box with a web-like bottom on which powdered moxa is placed. When the herb is burned, the box warms up. Held over the treatment area, it allows a diffuse and less intense heat to influence the flow of *qi* in a larger segment of the body. Moxa on needles, used mainly in Korean and Japanese acupuncture, involves the placing of a small cone of moxa at the end of a needle. As it is set alight, the needle heats up and has increased impact on the *qi*.

Moxa is dominantly used to tonify and stimulate *qi*-flow as well as to expel cold and dampness. It smells rather like marijuana and creates a fairly intensive smoke, which also tends to linger in clothes. For this reason, although it is a highly efficient way of treatment, it is received with some reserve by Westerners who prefer smokeless forms of moxa or TDP lamps. In East Asia, on the other hand, moxa is used commonly, not only by practitioners but also by the patients themselves. Readily available do-it-yourself kits provide small home-use cones, where the herb is placed in a tiny cylinder placed on a round base, which in turn has a sticky bottom for adherence to the skin. These cones never burn directly down to the skin and give some relief to colds and muscle aches.

The modern explanation for the efficacy of moxibustion is that it is a heat-transfer medium, but the traditional view sees it as vibratory stimulation, like rubbing or stroking. While nearly all acupuncture points are available for needling, quite a few are not indicated for moxibustion. The textbooks will in each case specify whether or not a point is recommended for moxa treatment or should be avoided (see www.acuxo.com; www.yinyanghouse.com). To treat a given disorder, the acupuncturist after establishing a diagnosis, has to decide which points to treat and in which manner. To select a point, various guidelines are offered.

First there are *local* points, near the area of pain or symptoms. A good example is LI-20 at the side of the nostrils for nasal congestion. Next, there are *remote* or distal points, located on the meridian associated with the disorder but at a distance, most commonly below the elbow or knee. Examples here are St-36 on the lower leg and or Lv-3 on top of the foot. Third, there are *symptomatic* points, chosen not because they are close to the pain or on the same meridian but because they work for the same kinds of symptoms. For example, LI-4 between thumb and index finger or LI-11 in the crease of the elbow may be chosen for their fever-reducing qualities even if the disease has nothing to do with the large intestine.

Another type is what might be called *theme points*, i.e., points that contain a similar name and work for similar disorders. A good example is a group of points that have to do with "wind," a major cause of disease. They are Wind Hall (GV-16), Wind Pond (Gb-20), Wind Gate (Bl-12), Wind Holder (St-12), Wind Protector (TH 17), and Wind Square (Gb-31). All except the last, which is located on the thigh, are found at the back of the head and around the neck and shoulders. Needling them in all cases controls wind after it has entered the body, having a releasing and warming effect. They are used to treat colds, paralysis, itches, joint pains, headaches, and vertigo (see Yao, "Ventus"). Another example is a set of three points that deal with "water": Water Ditch (GV-26), Water Division (CV-9), and Water Way (St-28). They are used to reduce swellings, help in cases of epilepsy, and enhance digestion, especially urination. Located in the face, abdomen, and lower torso respectively, they are also closely associated with the triple heater and open their respective body sections to the release of water (see Bai, "Wasser").

In addition, there is a set of twelve "spirit points" that all have the word *shen* in their name and are, with the exception of Spirit Gate (Ht-7) at the wrist, located on the head and torso. They are used to help with psycho-emotional problems that impair a patient's self-perception in the world, being either too caught in outside affairs or too focused on oneself (see Willmont, *Spirit Points*). A further set of thirteen "Ghost Points," which have the character *gui* (ghost) in their names was already defined in the Tang dynasty (618-907). They, too, are located for the most part on the torso and include Ghost Palace (GV-26), Ghost Bed (St-6), Ghost Heart (PC-7), and Ghost Path (Bl-62). Used traditionally for exorcism and cases of possession, they are nowadays activated to treat manic disorders and epilepsy (see Jarrett, *Clinical Practice*).

Beyond these theme points, there are also *combining* points, where several meridians flow together and whose treatment has an effect on a variety of channels. For example, Sp-6, three inches above the ankle on the inside leg, is called the Three Yin Interchange; it is a point on the spleen meridian at a spot where also the liver and kidney meridians run. The point maintains blood and *jing* and is also connected to the eight extraordinary vessels, thus creating a forum for broad-spectrum treatment. Similarly, GV-20, the Hundred Meeting point at the top of the head, is known for its "fivefold connection of three yang." That is to say, it is at a point through which also the small intestine, bladder, and gall bladder meridians run, the "three yang," and which intersects with the triple heater and the liver channels, creating a "fivefold connection." It is accordingly good for any number of conditions, especially wind-induced disorders such as colds, head-related problems, sensory issues, and various types of depletion.

Similarly broad-spectrum points are also found in the so-called eight *meeting points* or "influential points," each responsible for one particular aspect of the body: the yin-organs (Lv-13), the yang-organs (CV-12), the *qi* (CV-17), the blood (Bl-17), the sinews (Gb-34), the blood vessels (Lu-9), the bones (Bl-11), and the marrow (Gb-39). There are also four *dominant points*, each considered essential for treating a certain upper body region: stomach and abdomen (St-36), back (Bl-40), head and neck (Lu-7), and face and mouth (LI-4). There are further classifications of this sort for the lower parts of the body and in other modes of division, each selected for efficacy and practicality by individual acupuncturists.

A different way of selecting points is by examining the specific nature of the point within the pattern of the meridian in question. For example, each meridian has a *source point*, located near the wrist or ankle, where the source *qi* of the channel flows and where it is retained and strengthened most easily. The source point of the lung meridian is Lu-9, that of the liver meridian Lv-3, that of the gall bladder channel Gb-40. Then there are also so-called *alarm points*, located on the chest and abdomen where the *qi* of each meridian tends to gather, and whose palpitation gives direct access to the *qi* in the organ. They include Lu-1 for the lung, Lv-14 for the liver, and Gb-24 for the gall bladder. These are preferred points for activating or dispersing *qi* in the channels.

To make matters even more complex, there are also points associated with each of the five phases on all the meridians. They are known as the *five transport points* because they are responsible for pushing and moving the *qi* along. Located at the extremities, they tend to be the first or last points in a given meridian. They are described as the well point, where the *qi* originates; the gushing point where it begins to flow; the transporting point where the flow deepens; the traversing point where the *qi* flows vigorously; and the uniting point where it converges — each associated with the productive cycle of the five phases (Chen and Wang, *Acupuncture Case Histories*, 8).

To treat with these points, acupuncturists identify the location of the problem in terms of the meridians and of the productive cycle of the five phases. This means that if someone has a bladder problem that is also related to the liver, the two phases under consideration are water and wood. To treat the problem, the water point on the wood channel (Lv-11), could be needled; or the wood point on the water channel (Bl-65). This mode of point selection is expressed in terms of a "mother-son" relationship, wood being the child or "son" of water in the productive cycle. "For deficiency tonify the mother; for excess, drain the son" (*Difficult Issues*, ch. 69). To enhance treatment by giving it more of a single focus, one could also needle the water point on the water channel (Bl-66) or the wood point on the wood meridian (Lv-1).

> **Exercise:** Select a condition you are familiar with and identify three suitable acupuncture points. Decide what kind of needle to use, how to insert it, and for how long you would leave it to achieve optimal treatment.

Every practitioner learns these different points and modes in acupuncture school, then in active practice finds his or her best venue for treatment, and over time relies increasingly on experience and intuition. Two equally competent acupuncturists may accordingly disagree widely as to the preferred mode of treatment, and yet they may both be successful. Nor would this be anything new; in fact, some of the major divisions among acupuncture schools in history have been related to this issue.

To give one example, in the Yuan-dynasty of the thirteenth century, there were four great schools that each rested on a different premise for treatment and none of which was obviously better or more efficacious than the other (see Despeux, "Geschichte"). The four schools were: the Cooling School founded by Liu Wansu (1110-1200), which saw the cause of most ailments in a chronic state of inflammation due to the rising of inner fire and treated mainly by increasing the water in the kidneys; the Purgative School of Zhang Congzheng (1150-1228), which identified a variety of pathogens (e.g., wind, heat, dryness, dew, rain, ice, and dirt) that had to be eliminated before proper *qi*-flow could be achieved and accordingly strove to get rid of them as vigorously as possible, mainly by inducing sweating, vomiting, and diarrhea; the Earth Tonifying School of Li Gao (1180-1251), which saw the stomach and spleen as the main entryway of *qi* and thus central for healing, and treated mainly by strengthening earth meridians and earth points; and finally the Yin Moisturizing School founded by Zhu Zhenheng (1281-1358), which claimed that all yin tended toward deficiency and all yang toward excess, located the origin of diseases in the lack of yin-*qi* due to sexual and emotional activity, and focused on supporting the body's yin-moisture through enhancing the kidneys and other yin channels.

The wide disparity in modes of diagnosis and treatment within acupuncture, however, does not mean that needling any odd acupuncture point or administering any sort of treatment will have the desired effect. It just indicates that the body's energy system is complex and intricate and can be accessed in different ways, and that treatments become more efficient as they are tailored more precisely to the needs and patterns of the individual. Still, certain standard patterns remain, so that "wind" points are highly suitable for the common cold, spleen meridian points help to balance menstruation, and heart points most closely affect psychological states. The more detailed and intricate the point selection, moreover, the more efficient the treatment, and some of the more proficient acupuncturists pride themselves in using only two or three points per patient in any one session, localizing the exact lever for the patient's condition with great precision.

Further Readings

Bai, Liangchuan. 1999. "Zur 'Wasser'-ausleitenden Wirkung der drei Foramina 'Shui'." *Chinesische Medizin* 3/1999: 90-96.

Chen, Jirui, and Nissi Wang, eds. 1988. *Acupuncture Case Histories from China.* Seattle: Eastland Press.

Despeux, Catherine. 2000-02. "Geschichte der chinesischen Medizin." *Chinesische Medizin* 1/2000-3/2002 (10 parts).

Engelhardt, Ute. 1998. "Neue archäologische Funde zur Leitbahntheorie." *Chinesische Medizin* 3/1998: 93-100.

Harper, Donald. 1999. *Early Chinese Medical Manuscripts: The Mawangdui Medical Manuscripts.* London: Wellcome Asian Medical Monographs.

Jarrett, Lonny S. 2003. *The Clinical Practice of Chinese Medicine.* Stockbridge, Mass.: Spirit Path Press.

Ki, Sunu. 1985. *The Canon of Acupuncture: Huangti Nei Ching Ling Shu.* Los Angeles: Yuin University Press.

Kuriyama, Shigehisa. 1999. *The Expressiveness of the Body and the Divergence of Greek and Chinese Medicine.* New York: Zone Books.

Lu, Gwei-djen. 1980. *Celestial Lancets: A History and Rationale of Acupuncture and Moxa.* Cambridge: Cambridge University Press.

Lu, Henry C. 1987. *The Yellow Emperor's Book of Acupuncture.* Blaine, Wash.: Academy of Oriental Heritage.

Ni, Maoshing. 1995. *The Yellow Emperor's Classic of Medicine.* Boston: Shambhala.

Unschuld, Paul U. 1986. *Nan-ching: The Classic of Difficult Issues.* Berkeley: University of California Press.

_____. 2000. *Medicine in China: Historical Artifacts and Images.* New York: Prestel.

Veith, Ilza. 1972. *The Yellow Emperor's Classic of Internal Medicine.* Berkeley: University of California Press.

Willmont, Dennis. 2001. *The Twelve Spirit Points of Acupuncture.* Marshfield, Mass.: Willmountain Press.

Wu, Jing-Nuan. 1993. *Ling Shu or The Spiritual Pivot.* Washington, D.C.: The Taoist Center.

Yao, Yufang. 2000. "Die 'Ventus'-Foramina." *Chinesische Medizin* 2/2000: 39-47.

Chapter 8
Forms of Massage

Massage is another form of Chinese clinical health practice. It involves the systematic manipulation of the body's soft tissue, i.e., muscles, tendons, and fascia, with the goal of promoting relaxation, reducing tension, relieving stress, and alleviating ailments. Massage has been known throughout human history and presumably began when early cave dwellers rubbed each other's aches. The ancient Greeks describe it in their medical books, and the Romans were very fond of it. Julius Caesar had himself rubbed and pinched regularly for neuralgia, while the Roman naturalist Pliny received massages to control asthma. Modern Western massage began with the work of Per Henrik Ling of Sweden (1776-1839). A fencing master and avid exerciser, he developed a system that mixed medical gymnastics and massages to cure himself of rheumatism. His method, which consists largely of rhythmical deep-tissue stroking, became popular and was later codified and taught at the Royal Gymnastics Central Institute in Stockholm. Known as Swedish massage, it is still the standard Western treatment (www.massageandbodywork.com; www.amta.org).

Chinese massage has been recorded since ancient times. Clearly mentioned in the *Yellow Emperor's Inner Classic*, it has appeared as a major medical specialization in medical manuals since the Tang (618-907). Not merely for pain relief and relaxation, massage in China is an effective and comprehensive form of clinical therapy, closely related to acupuncture in its use of the meridian system and diagnostic techniques. Applied to many health problems, it seeks to establish a harmonious flow of *qi* and to encourage the body to heal itself. It also forms an important part of Daoist practice, especially as self-massages that stimulate *qi*.

Massage can be undertaken informally among friends or couples or can be provided professionally by a trained therapist. In all cases, it should be practiced in a quiet, clean environment with enough leisure to afford good relaxation. The giver should make sure to have clean, warm hands and short fingernails and should not wear any rings or bracelets that might hurt or disturb the receiver. There needs to be a mental harmony between giver and receiver, since the will to heal becomes manifest in the strokes of the hands. While the giver wears loose, comfortable clothing to feel most at ease, in many forms of Western massage the receiver undresses completely and is covered with a loose sheet. The skin is treated directly, often with the help of some lubricant to ease friction. However, it is not necessary for the receiver to be in the nude: and many forms of Eastern massage are given through light clothing without lubrication or they focus to a large extent on the extremities.

Most commonly in the West, and also in China nowadays, the patient lies on a massage table and the practitioner stands. In India, Thailand, and Japan, however, the patient is on the floor and the massage therapist kneels or sits in various positions, moving around the patient. The floor position has the advantage that in addition to finger pressure, the weight of the entire body can be used. Some Western practices, notably Rolfing, also make use of other pressures than fingers, using wrists, elbows, and knees to manipulate specific areas. At the other end of the massage spectrum are techniques that apply no pressure at all, but are a form of the laying-on of hands. Resting the hands on a particular body part, or even holding them above it, the practitioner channels cosmic healing energy into the patient. In the U.S., this form is best known as therapeutic touch; it appears both in Japanese Reiki and in Chinese Qigong.

When hands are used, massage applies a number of classical strokes. Since these were first classified in nineteenth-century Europe, they have names based on French terms. They are:

1. effleurage—stroking of the skin: can be a deep stroke to stimulate tissue and to force fluids to move into a certain direction; a lighter, slow stroke used for relaxation; or a light, fast stroke to stimulate blood flow;

2. petrissage—lifting and kneading of the skin: stretches and separates muscle fiber, fascia, and scar tissue;

3. friction—deep pressure: mobilizes muscles and separates tissue, including the breakup of scar tissue;

4. tapotement—tapping or pounding the skin: used for relaxation and desensitization of nerve endings, as well as to break up congestion in certain organs (e.g., lungs);

5. vibration—rapid shaking of tissue: increases blood flow and provides systemic invigoration.

A massage can last from fifteen minutes to several hours and can be administered for a variety of problems. Most common in the West are muscle aches and pains, sports injuries, and the loosening of scar tissue. Massages should not be given without a proper diagnosis and clear purpose. If the patient has a heart, lung, or kidney problem, atherosclerosis, varicose veins, or other chronic conditions, these need to be taken into consideration. Also, while performing the massage, the practitioner must never press on an open wound, swelling, or an area of infection or inflamed skin. She should avoid direct pressure on lymph nodes, bruised areas, fresh scars, varicose veins, and areas of fractures. To be properly ready for a massage, it is best not to have taken alcohol for a day and not to have a full stomach. Massages are also less effective when received immediately after a hot bath, after strenuous exercise, or in states of extreme fatigue. Special care has to be taken during pregnancy. After the massage it is best to rest for ten to fifteen minutes to get the full effect.

> **Exercise:** Reach out and touch someone. Now, reach out and touch someone with a warm, caring thought in your mind. Find a sensitive area and touch it, using the various strokes and maintaining an awareness of healing and giving. Feel the difference in your mind and fingers.

The physiological effect of a whole-body massage is manifold. It activates the immune system, assists the venous flow of blood, enhances the lymphatic flow, stretches the muscles and enhances their oxygenation. It also can loosen scar tissue and increase the metabolism by moving the muscles, allowing them to release acids into the lymphatic and venous flow. This effect carries over into a general sense of well-being and a release of stress and tension. People who receive massages regularly tend to be less tired and easier to live with; they are healthier and lead more balanced lives.

There are two major forms of massage in China: Anmo and Tuina. Anmo, literally "press and rub," is an expanded form of acupressure. While acupressure is the manipulation of acupuncture points with fingers rather than needles, Anmo goes beyond the main meridians and also makes use of the extraordinary vessels and the muscular system. It is used for health maintenance and healing as well as in Qigong. Exerting pressure through fingers and palms, it aims to give a balanced full-body treatment, combining yang techniques of expelling stagnant *qi* and activating flow with yin practices of calming and relaxing. It does not apply oils or other lubricants and can be done through clothing, while the patient is either sitting up or lying down.

The practitioner, after examining the patient and reaching a diagnosis, stimulates key points on the body surface to promote its healing abilities and increase circulation. Anmo is flexible in style and can be used any-time and anywhere. Its overall effects are to balance the body, calm the nerves, normalize body functions, increase strength, reduce tension, and effect rejuvenation. It is quite popular and typically used for everyday discomforts (see *acupuncture.com*). Examples of points to be manipulated for common problems include:

> Headache: GB-20 (neck), GB-34 (upper calf), LI-4 (thumb), Lv-3 (top of foot, near ankle), St-36 (below the knee);
>
> Menstrual problems: GB-21 (above neck), LI-4 (thumb), Sp-6 (three inches above the ankle), St-36 (below the knee);
>
> Cold: GB-20 (neck), LI-4 (thumb), LI-20 (side of nose), Lv-3 (top of foot);
>
> Nausea: St 36 (below the knee), PC 6 (above the wrist).

One subcategory of Anmo has grown into a separate tradition: foot and hand massage. It follows the ancient Chinese belief that the extremities are microcosms of the body and are central in manipulating the meridi-ans. While traditional Anmo practitioners also treat hands and feet, the idea here is that massaging fingers, toes, palms, and soles alone has a sufficient effect on the internal organs to create health and vigor.

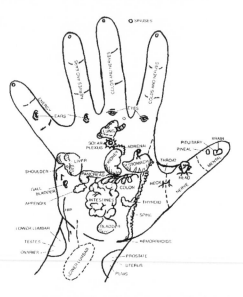

This idea is not limited to China, but is also documented in ancient Egypt and among Native Americans. In the West, it is known as reflexology and began as "zone therapy" in 1913 when William Fitzgerald identified ten symmetrical, longitudinal zones linking nerve endings and organs with the hands and feet, so that the entire body is reflected.

Fig. 16. The reflex zones on the hand.

Thus on the foot, the reflexology points for the head are in the toes, those for neck and throat at their root, those for chest and stomach in the balls of the feet, those for liver, gall bladder, and intestines on the soles, and those for lower pelvis, hips, and legs at the heel. The same pattern applies also to the hands, where the head matches the fingers and the torso is spread over the palm and wrists (www.aboutreflexology.com).

Hands and feet are manipulated with a variety of techniques. Gripping involves the fingers of one hand producing pressure while the thumb and palm of the other reinforce and stabilize the object. Rotation is the twisting of joints in either toes or fingers, usually held between two fingers and the thumb. Walking means that the thumb and fingers walk over an entire sole or palm. Rubbing involves the exertion of steady pressure along the tendon lines on top of the feet or hands. Rolling, finally, can be done with a golf ball or other round object that is moved back and forth over the feet or hands to exert pressure. Typically no creams, oils, or herbs are used in a given session, which may last between fifteen and forty-five minutes. The entire foot or hand is treated first, then time is spent on particular problem areas. It can also be self-administered, and holistic practitioners recommend massaging the feet daily for maintaining internal health (www.reflexology-usa.net).

> **Exercise:** Find the pressure points of the main organs and body parts on your hand. Massage them. See how you feel.

The other major form of Chinese massage is Tuina, which literally means "push and grasp." Somewhat like Western chiropractic and naprapathic practices, it involves the manipulation of joints and bones as much as the massage of muscles and tissues. Tuina helps with injuries, internal disorders, and skeletal problems. Its moves, include pressing with the thumbs, palms, fists, balls of the hands, and elbows; grasping by pulling up tissues with the thumb and fingers; rolling the flesh with the back of the hand; kneading by manipulating the muscles with fingers and rolling them in circular moves; as well as rotation for joints and stretches for myofascial tissue.

Tuina makes use both of the traditional meridian system and of the muscle and bone structure of the body. Using deep-tissue manipulation and joint work, it can be painful as it realigns anatomical structures, releases spasms, relaxes tissues, opens adhesions, and lubricates the joints. Making people sweat, it expels cold pathological factors and regulates the *qi* (see www.acupuncture.com; www.planetherbs.com/articles/tuina.html).

These classical methods of Chinese massage were also adopted into Japan, where three major methods have evolved. The oldest is Shiatsu, which literally means "finger pressure." It was adapted first by Japanese Buddhist monks who visited China in the ninth century C.E. to collect Buddhist teachings and also brought back medical texts and methods. As an independent form of health care, Shiatsu goes back to the early twentieth century and today comes in three major forms: Shiatsu massage, which sees the body largely from an anatomical perspective and makes use of muscle and nerve structures (Namikoshi 1981); acupressure which follows the Chinese meridian model (Serizawa 1984); and Zen Shiatsu which recognizes a broader set of meridians and uses a lighter level of pressure (Masunaga and Ohashi 1977).

Typically Shiatsu is practiced on the floor with the patient fully clothed. Besides fingers and hands, it uses three or four fingers, elbows, knees, and feet. The strokes are executed rhythmically and come in many different forms — pressing, hooking, sweeping, shaking, rotating, grasping, vibrating, patting, plucking, lifting, pinching, rolling, and brushing. The four major hand positions are palm, i.e., the entire palm is pressed on the face, back, abdomen, or legs to provide a soft stimulation of wider areas; heel of hand, i.e., with *qi* focused on the heel of the hand, the practitioner applies strong, steady pressure; fingers, i.e., holding a limb or section between fingers and thumb, a strong pressure is applied, while the practitioner visualizes the *qi* in the patient's body; and thumb, i.e., pressing the thumbs supported by the other four fingers deeply into the tissue.

Different types of pressure include a sustained push with the whole body weight behind it, a continuous steady exertion to infuse healing *qi*, and a perpendicular pressure exerted vertically with extended arms. Even then, the practitioner should never look down at the hands but keep an upright posture to maintain smooth *qi*-flow. In the beginning students learn the sequence and location of points as well as the hand positions and pressures mechanically, but later they become intuitive more meditative in their practice. Shiatsu has been found effective for cramps, headaches, fatigue, and poor circulation; it also promotes concentration, focus, balance, and coordination and aids the body's own healing (see www.shiatsu.org).[1]

---

[1] An American adaptation of Shiatsu in conjunction with acupressure was developed by Dennis Willmont and Barbara Blanchard, combining both in yin-yang

A second, more modern adaptation of Chinese massage in Japan is Jinshindo, literally the "Way of the Compassionate Heart." Formulated in the U.S. by Iona Teeguarden, it is based on Anmo techniques of acupressure and uses select points from both the main meridians and the extraordinary vessels, using a basic set of thirty and an advanced set of forty-five. The practice applies pressure on specific points for prolonged periods, often combining a local point where the symptom is most obvious with a distal one, located at the far end of the same meridian. The idea is that these acupuncture points are containers of traumatic memories and emotional tensions. The points are, moreover, located in specific segments of the body, each associated with a particular form of psychological tension, so that, for example, the neck is linked with a division between the rational and feeling parts of the body and with the choking down of feelings, while the chest is the seat of restricted and suppressed emotions. Often common clichés give an indication of the mind-body relationship addressed.

Exercise: Think of some common clichés using the body to describe personal problems or tendencies, such as "pain in the neck," "no guts," and the like. How are they possibly related to physical symptoms and conditions?

A classic set of points for the basic neck release uses five points on either side of the neck and shoulders, combining points of the gallbladder, triple heater, and small intestine meridians and numbering them in a special Jinshido way (nos. 19-23).

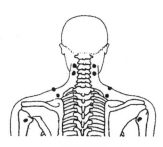

Another common pattern holds Lu-1 on the inside of the shoulder with one hand while pressing Lu-10 at the base of the thumb with the other.

Fig. 17. Points for basic neck release.

As the *qi* flows more smoothly, the patient will feel a pulsation in the points and a release of physical and psychological pressure. Iona Teeguarden tells the story of a young woman named Mary who had been told all her life not to be a weepy wimp. She suffered from asthma and the inability to express sadness and anxiety. Instead she tended to

---

polarity and making use of all meridians and acupuncture points. For details, see www.willmountain.com.

give vent to massive explosions of rage. Applying pressure to the points on the lung meridian and suggesting that the patient give herself permission to cry, much of the armored tension was released and her asthma receded (*Jin Shin Do Handbook*, 8). The practice can also be self-administered, using for example Gb-20 at the base of the neck and Gb-14 above the eyebrow to relieve headaches.

A third form of Japanese massage is Reiki, literally "numinous *qi*," the channeling of cosmic life force through the practitioner into the patient. It goes back to the mid-nineteenth century when Mikao Usui, a Christian minister in search of the Buddha's and Jesus' healing methods, underwent a three-week fast on Mount Kurama near Kyoto and received the power to heal. After developing in Japan, Reiki was spread to the U.S. in 1937 by Ms. Hawayo Takata of Hawai'i and has been flourishing ever since. Today practitioners train in weekend seminars to achieve several levels of attunement and healing activation.

Reiki practitioners lay-on hands on specific entry spots to affect the entire body. Instead of curing, they stimulate the innate healing ability of the body. Enhancing energy and balance and giving the receiver a sense of serenity and strength, it helps with multiple illnesses, injuries, and psychological issues. It can also decrease the side effects of drugs and chemotherapy and is used by practitioners in mutual sessions to strengthen their immune system and prevent diseases (www.reikicare.co.uk).

Reiki is done either sitting up or lying down, and practitioners learn twelve key positions on the head, front, and back of the body. It is also possible to heal at a distance by sending healing cosmic *qi* to the person in question—not unlike the work of prayer groups in certain Christian circles. Reiki emphasizes a pure state of mind and encourages practitioners to begin treatments by placing their hands together and visualize a white light passing through their body, thinking loving thoughts, and repeating the five basic principles of the teaching:

> Just for today, do not worry.
> Just for today, do not anger.
> Just for today, do an honest day's work.
> Just for today, be grateful for all life's blessings.
> Just for today, be kind to every living being. (Klinger-Omenka,
> *Reiki*, 19; see also www.reiki.org; reiki.7gen.com).

Similar to Reiki is a form of contemporary Chinese Qigong, known as external *qi* healing. Here, too, the practitioner becomes a channel for the universal life force. Although the most common setting is formal treatments as in acupuncture or massage, there is ultimately no need for them, and even casual contact, such as shaking hands or directing intention, will have the desired effect.

It takes some Qigong practice to reach the level of external *qi* healing. Practitioners should practice regularly until the *qi*-flow in their bodies is strong and steady and they have some control over it. Only then can the *qi* be directed outward for healing. In a *qi* healing session the practitioner holds her hands about six inches above the patient's body and allows the *qi* to arrive. The attitude is one of well-wishing and peace, openness, nonaction, and softness—prime virtues in ancient Daoism. As the hands keep steady, *qi* disperses or increases; as they move along the meridians, *qi* begins to flow. The therapeutic range is the same as for acupuncture and massage: it can reduce pain, shrink swellings, eliminate cancer cells, ease arthritis, release tension, and help with many other conditions (see Jahnke, *Healer Within*).

The practice of external *qi* healing goes back far into Chinese history and can be linked with shamans of old. It was also commonly known among medieval Daoists, who actively spread *qi* to others as their own became replete. To nourish their *qi*, they practiced gymnastics, breathing exercises, and meditations: loosening the muscles, opening the pathways, and concentrating the mind. Another way in which Daoists encouraged the development of external *qi* was by using techniques of self-massage, which is another dimension of Chinese massage practice that survives today.

Self-massage can be like reflexology and focus on the feet, hands, and ears; it can also center on specific areas, stroking, kneading, or holding points in a painful or obstructed part of the body; or it can be a gentle systematic stroking of the entire body. For example:

> Start by rubbing your hands together until they feel warm. Then, as if you were washing your face, pass your hands upward—starting at the neck and chin and then over the cheeks, eyes, and forehead. Pass your hands over the top of the head, down the back of the neck, and along the shoulders as if you were bathing in a powerful healing resource. Bring the hands around the front of the shoulders, under the arms and reach around the back and up as high on the back as possible. Continue down the back, over the sacrum, and down the backs of the legs. . . .

Then come around to the front and inside the legs and pass the hands upward along the torso to begin again with the face. Imagine you are standing in a pool of healing waters. As your hands come around, imagine you are gathering from this pool handfuls of a marvelous healing elixir and bathing yourself with it from top to bottom. (Jahnke, *Healer Within*, 71-72)

Exercise: Follow the above instructions. How do you feel after a session?

Like all other forms of massages, self-massage involves guiding the *qi* along the lines of the meridians. Practicing it regularly keeps the *qi* circulating, the body healthy, and the mind at peace.

Further Readings

Beck, Mark F. 1994. *Theory and Practice of Therapeutic Massage*. Albany: Milady.

Gach, Michael Reed, with Carolyn Marco. 1981. *Acu-Yoga: Self Help Techniques to Relieve Tension*. New York: Japan Publications.

Jahnke, Roger. 1997. *The Healer Within Using Traditional Chinese Techniques to Release Your Body's Own Medicine*. San Francisco: HarperCollins.

Klinger-Omenka, Ursula. 1997. *Reiki with Gemstones*. Twin Lakes, Wis.: Lotus Light.

Masunaga, Shizuto, and Wataru Ohashi. 1977. *Zen Shiatsu*. New York: Japan Publications.

Namikoshi, Tokujiro. 1981. *The Complete Book of Shiatsu Therapy*. New York: Japan Publications.

Serizawa, Katsusuke. 1976. *Effective Tsubo Therapy*. New York: Japan Publications.

Sohn, Tina, and Robert Sohn. 1996. *Amma Therapy: A Complete Textbook of Oriental Bodywork and Medical Principles*. Rochester, Vt.: Healing Arts Press.

Stein, Diane. 1996. *Essential Reiki: A Complete Guide to an Ancient Healing Art*. Freedom, Calif.: The Crossing Press.

Tappan, Frances M. 1988. *Healing Massage Techniques: Holistic, Classic, and Emerging Methods*. Norwalk: Appleton & Lange.

Teeguarden, Iona. 1991. *Jin Shin Do Handbook*. Idyllwild, Calif.: Jin Shin Do Foundation.

Chapter 9
Medicine in China Today

In China today, Eastern and Western medical systems are increasingly integrated, while attitudes toward traditional medicine change in accordance with trends in government policies. They can be characterized by two major underlying themes: nationalism and public health care.

Medicine was drafted into a nationalist agenda from the earliest appearance of Western biomedicine in the sixteenth century, when the Catholic missionary Matteo Ricci arrived in China. Under the Qing dynasty, the Kangxi emperor (r. 1662-1722) favored Western physicians, since he was cured by missionaries of his malaria attacks. He established the first Western-style hospital at the imperial court and encouraged the integration of Western anatomy and pharmacology into the Chinese system.

The Western impact, however, did not reach into the larger populace where traditional practice continued to dominate. The people regarded Western medical knowledge with great suspicion, exacerbated by the fact that Western science and technology came to them with military conquest and colonization. As the Chinese became more hostile to westernization, traditional medicine was praised as a bulwark of traditional learning that bolstered nationalist pride and cultural identity in the face of invasive foreign forces.

While this attitude changed after the fall of the Qing dynasty and the foundation of the Chinese Republic in 1911, a very similar nationalist agenda elevating Chinese medicine as a positive force in Chinese identity appeared again in the early years of the People's Republic. In the 1950s, Mao Zedong found it necessary to create his own brand of third-world Communism, clearly distinct from the Russian model. Although against all superstition and feudalistic practices with which medicine had often been linked, he elevated acupuncture and related techniques to a positive factor in the uniqueness of the Chinese experience and greatly supported its practice. Under his augury the first colleges in Chinese medicine were established in 1956, setting the stage for its development under state control.

The nationalist perspective on Chinese medicine did not only have a positive and supporting effect, however. Another way in which nationalism impacted on its understanding was by seeing it as a major obstacle to modernization and the full acceptance of China among the world's leaders. In this vision, nationalism was not served by emphasizing Chinese uniqueness and ancient traditions. On the contrary, nationalist realization could only be attained by abolishing all ancient and outdated ways, making China a modern country and proving Chinese superiority by competing with Western nations on their own turf.

The leadership of China's first republican government, which came to power under the Kuomintang party in 1911, was the strongest representative of this view. Sun Yat-sen and many other leaders studied abroad to learn Western science and medicine with only minimal knowledge of the traditional ways. Generally opposed to East Asian medical practice, the Kuomintang supported a proposal for its complete abolition, which passed initial approval by the Chinese Ministry of Health in 1929. It severely restricted the practice of Chinese medicine, prohibited all advertising for traditional techniques, and prevented the establishment of colleges.

While this measure was never implemented due to massive protests of practitioners and patients, a similar attitude toward Chinese medicine has prevailed in the People's Republic since 1949, with the brief exception of the 1950s. The dominant view, governed by dialectical materialism, has been that all traditional ideas and practices, and especially those that involve spiritual or supernatural concepts, are saturated with feudalism and superstition and need to be extirpated ruthlessly. Chinese medicine is allowed to survive because of its unique contribution to the revolution—and the forbidding cost of Western medicine—but it cannot remain as it was. It has to be "modernized," made acceptable in Western scientific and biomedical terms.

This modernization began in the 1960s. It meant that traditional doctors, commonly trained in a hands-on apprenticeship system, had to undergo scientific training and formal college education. They had to study Western sciences—biology, chemistry, anatomy, and so on—in order to be fully equivalent to Western-trained physicians. It also meant that healing procedures and herbal remedies were to be tested formally in clinical trials, with double-blind studies and animal experiments. The language of Chinese medicine, moreover, was altered to increasingly include biomedical terms, seeing the body more and more as a mechanism and focusing on the identification of diseases rather than on seeing the patient in a larger context. This modernized version of Chinese medicine is called "Traditional Chinese Medicine" or TCM. It is quite different from the practice as described in the ancient textbooks. It is also more the result of political demands than an organic development of the tradition.

So much for the nationalist agenda. The other major framework for the practice of medicine in China today is public health care. The idea of public health care arose in the nineteenth century, mainly in England and Germany, when medical research made it clear that nutrition, hygiene, and inoculation could significantly reduce infant mortality and the outbreak of epidemics. Entire cities were restructured to allow the installation of proper sewage systems; vaccines, first for smallpox, later for tuberculosis, were made available to large portions of the population; and fresh fruit and unspoiled bread were lauded as aiding health and survival.

Unlike in earlier centuries when health care had been the domain of the family and village, building a sewage system and managing mass inoculations required the organizational clout of an overarching authority. The budding nation states of Europe accordingly took it upon themselves to undertake the necessary measures and created appropriate bureaucracies, such as local and national boards of health. Public health care became a task of the state. In due course the state was seen as responsible for the well-being of its citizens, the key authority to tell people how to live, what to eat, and where to turn in case of illness.

The late nineteenth and early twentieth centuries saw the expansion of these ideas into the international arena. The driving force behind this was the increasing trade with other nations and the colonies. Lesser developed countries did not practice the same health care measures as the Europeans and accordingly exported disease together with tea, gold, and spices. Several major international conferences were convened on questions of sanitation to create general guidelines and international standards. Nothing much came of them, however, until after World War I, when the League of Nations formed a supranational health care agency that installed suitable measures.

The Chinese public health care system was directly influenced by the measures proposed by the League of Nations. That a centralized system of medicine was needed had become painfully clear when a pneumonic plague ravaged northeastern China in 1910-11. Accordingly, in the 1920s, after the civil war surrounding the fall of the Qing, various administrative measures were put into place, including the establishment of regional boards of health and a central Ministry of Health. By 1949, when the Communists came to power, the idea that the state ran the health care system and was responsible for the well-being of its citizens had been firmly entrenched. Since then, every Chinese has been automatically insured through the National Health Service, and all doctors, nurses, and medical workers have been—at least until very recently—state employees and public servants, controlled in a highly complex bureaucratic system. The end of private medical practice standardized health services, but it also severely limited the freedom of traditional practitioners, destroyed innovation and independence, and increased the need for other health support. It thus contributed significantly to the boom in alternative health techniques, such as Qigong and Taiji quan.

	Government	
	State Council	
National Ministry of Higher Education		National Ministry of Public Health
	Academy of Medical Sciences	
	Specialized Hospitals and Affiliated Medical Colleges	
Provincial Hospitals	Provincial Medical Schools	Health Departments
Municipal Hospitals		Health Bureaus
Factory Health Stations		
Street Health Stations		
Lane Health Substations		
Maternal and Child Care	District Hospitals	Health Bureaus
	Commune Clinics	
	Brigade Health Stations	
	Village Health Stations	
	Team Health Care Worker	

Fig. 18. The organization of Chinese public health services.

Exercise: Consider the health care system in your country and evaluate it in terms of universal coverage, effectiveness, and the role of alternative treatments. How is it different from the Chinese? What is better? What is worse?

During the Cultural Revolution in 1966-1976 health care was once again reorganized by the state. In June 1965, Mao Zedong published a set of notes, criticizing the Ministry of Health. He stated that too much emphasis was placed on urban health care and not enough on helping the population in the countryside, where still 80 percent of the population lived; curative medicine was given too high a priority, while preventive measures were not implemented effectively; too much emphasis was placed on Western medicine, which was not sufficiently integrated with traditional practices; there was still too much copying of models from other countries, especially the Soviet Union, rather than reliance on the wisdom of the people and the use of indigenous methods; the medical establishment was too much entrenched in a tight, hierarchical structure despite the value of collective leadership; there was too great an emphasis on raising the standards of health care instead of widening its accessibility; and last but not least, there was too much inbreeding and policy making among the managers who were not in touch with the people.

To remedy these ills, Mao proposed to take measures in three areas:

> Education: Three years in medical school are enough; students should continue study by practicing.
>
> Research: Fewer men and materials should be devoted to the "pinnacles of medicine," the complex and difficult diseases, and more to commonly occurring illnesses, the "urgent problems of the masses."
>
> Service: All doctors, unless of little experience or "lacking in ability," should be sent to the countryside to practice. (see Lucas, *Chinese Medical Modernization*)

As a result, medical education, both Western and Eastern, was cut short and numerous doctors were released into clinical practice without being fully trained. Countryside practitioners who had only rudimentary knowledge began to treat people, working as "barefoot doctors." Numerous city dwellers were sent into the country to "learn from the people," and primitive and often problematic methods of treatment were brought forward. Beyond all this, the people believed that revolutionary doctrines and the Chairman's sayings would cure all ills and that the country's health problems would evaporate with the extirpation of feudalistic thinking. Thus, for example, a 1968 article in *China's Medicine*, the official organ of the Chinese Medical Association, is entitled: "Mao Zedong's Thought Restores Vision to the Blind: Traditional Cataractopiesis in the Countryside." Ideology superseded all practical and clinical considerations.

In 1978, after the ousting of the Gang of Four and the rise of Deng Xiaoping to prime minister, these measures were reversed with the goal to bring China into the twentieth century and modernize with full speed. The so-called Four Modernizations became the leading doctrine of government, enhancing westernization and progress in the areas of industry, agriculture, science and technology, and the military. In terms of medical practice, this meant the establishment of plural health care, i.e., the offering of three basic alternatives through the public health care system: Chinese, Western, and integrated. Four new policies appeared:

1. A greater emphasis was placed on hospital-based services rather than primary or community care.

2. Moves were initiated toward the renewed professionalization of medicine, so that specialist knowledge came again to be valued above political correctness.

3. New developments were based on technology, including technology transfer from developed countries, both in tools and personnel.

4. Chinese and Western forms of medicine were to be treated as equal and should be integrated and merged.

Essentially, these policies are still in place today. Most patients are treated in hospitals rather than by independent practitioners; specialization has made great inroads both in Western and Chinese-style hospitals; technical data such as X-rays, blood pressure, and body temperature are commonplace; and patients have access to various forms of health care. Still, control lies to a great degree with the patient whose description of symptoms and health history determines the way the physician treats him or her. Typically, patients keep their own medical records in their "medical booklet" (*bingli ben*). They bring it to the clinic and hand it to the physician to note diagnosis and prescription. However, patients often lose their booklets and have to reconstruct their medical history from memory, making the system rather haphazard.

Chinese patients tend to make use of all the different modes of medical treatment. They often use both Western and Chinese prescriptions at the same time, undergo acupuncture or massage therapy while also taking antibiotics or preparing for surgery. An example is the case of a pediatric clinic in Chengdu, Sichuan. Physicians frequently over-prescribe antibiotics while also giving herbal formulas, thus promoting the antibiotic cycle of resistance that Western countries are trying to avoid. Patients appreciate this treatment, because the popular perception is that Western medicine acts fast, Chinese medicine slow; Western medicine treats ramifications, Chinese medicine the root; Western medicine often has side effects, Chinese medicine does not; and Western medicine is better for acute diseases, while Chinese medicine serves best in chronic cases. A line of treatment, therefore, may begin with some home remedies, turn to Western treatments for acute symptoms and ramifications, and—especially if it is not effective—move on to a Chinese cure for the root of the problem.

Exercise: Think about a medical condition or situation where multiple approaches may be justified or appropriate. Which Western and Eastern treatments might go well together? Which should not be mixed?

The multiplicity of medical care in China is also reflected in the way medicine is taught in the country. As studied by the British anthropologist Elisabeth Hsu in Kunming, Yunnan in 1988-89 and described in *The Transmission of Chinese Medicine*, there are three major venues in which Chinese medicine is transmitted: first, colleges of TCM with formal classes and a degree program; second, small study groups run by eminent elder physicians that read medical classics; and third, Qigong healers who accept apprentices on the basis of their natural talents and predestination.

Medical knowledge as transmitted in these three settings is widely divergent and taught in radically different styles. The greatest degree of standardization and systematization appears in the colleges, which provide proper accreditation. Traditional concepts are placed strongly into the modern framework of Western biomedicine and the Communist doctrine of dialectical materialism. Formal classroom instruction and rote memorization are the key activities of the students, who are often low in motivation since they did not choose this career from a strong inner urge but on the basis of family recommendations or because they were not accepted into a Western medical school.

Seminars led by learned elder doctors tend to focus on book learning and be highly authoritarian in structure. Students must memorize the original text and learn the master's particular interpretation, often idiosyncratic and based on free-style association rather than systematic exegesis. Some are very dedicated and memorize every word of the teacher, others—sent by their work unit or parents—do only the absolute minimum and often miss class. Unlike this, the setting with the Qigong master, although similarly authoritarian, is highly practical, teaching strictly by example. Each apprentice—carefully chosen, totally dedicated, and expected to work for many years—has to follow the master in all his movements, thereby learning basic hand gestures and Qigong patterns. The only verbal form of instruction is in Daoist chants that are mumbled to increase *qi*-potency, but they too are imitated and memorized. There are few explanations, and students are expected to absorb the teaching by practicing it in their bodies.

Taken together, these different modes of teaching Chinese medicine reflect the complexity of the system and show it as a rather disjointed jumble of ideas and practices. While the content may have some overlaps, such as the theory of five phases, and obviously the goal is similar in all, there is a strong discontinuity among them and even a sense of contradiction.

Certain key concepts, seen differently in the three venues, clarify this point. For example, *shen* or spirit plays a fairly significant role in Qigong healing, where often the symptoms do not change but the patient feels improved and is of better "spirit." In the learned readings, *shen* appears as a vague, rather nebulous concept, somehow linked with *qi* but generally ignored rather than explicated. In the modern college, finally, *shen* is increasingly left out of the curriculum—the classical triad of forces being changed from *jing, qi,* and *shen* in a textbook of 1984 to *jing, qi, xue* (blood), and *jinye* (body fluids) in 1988. Rather than acknowledging an indeterminate "spirit" component in healing, physicians prefer to follow a materialistic value system and use the factor phlegm (*tanyin*). Like *shen* it has a variety of functions and appearances, but is more tangible and can be seen, touched, and put under a microscope.

The effects of mechanizing and westernizing Chinese medicine are manifold. For one, practitioners increasingly diagnose in biomedical terms rather than along the lines of energetic patterns. Also, traditional syndromes, such as "blood stasis" are more and more identified by Western analogues, reducing the flexibility and intuitive power of the ancient system. Similarly, the curative effect of herbs is now understood as a chemical reaction rather than a complex energetic interrelation and subjected to clinical trials and animal experiments. This creates its own set of problems, since, as Judith Farquhar says in *Knowing Practice,* "the practical logic of Chinese medicine and its ways of seeking efficacy are thoroughly inconsistent with the epistemological strictures of the Western natural sciences."

A case in point is outlined by Heiner Fruehauf. It involves the testing of an herbal formula for easy childbirth prescribed successfully over generations by physicians in Chengdu, Sichuan. Subjected to animal experiments, it was injected into the uteri of rabbits with no effect whatsoever. Other substances found helpful in rabbits' births, on the other hand, had no benefits for humans. As Fruehauf comments,

> The elaborate procedures of a reductionist science can project a highly distorted picture of the reality of the human body. . . Rabbits, after all, are different from humans; human beings usually do not give birth in completely controlled conditions with their own uterus hanging from their bellies; and the remedy in question is designed to work via the digestive process of metabolic transformation. ("Science, Politics," 14)

It is thus not surprising that ways which have worked with people for generations cannot be proven in an isolated laboratory experiment, and that remedies found useful in a lab setting may or may not stand up in clinical practice. Also, traditional prescriptions were specifically tailored to the needs of the patients and cannot be easily applied in double-blind studies. Western analysis does not take that aspect of diagnosis and treatment into account, instead attempting to apply the same prescription to superficially similar symptoms.

TCM as practiced in China today is very different from the medicine of the classics, the dynamic medical traditions of imperial China, and its branches in other East Asian countries. It is no longer based on an integrated *qi*-based cosmology but follows scientific and materialist thinking; it no longer looks at the patient as a dynamic, complex whole but isolates symptoms and diseases; it is increasingly specialized and focused only on the body, losing the integrative vision of the patient as a social, emotional, and spiritual being; and it is more and more reduced to a technical skill rather than an intuitive art of healing.

Further Readings

Crozier, Ralph. 1968. *Traditional Medicine in Modern China: Science, Nationalism, and the Tensions of Cultural Change.* Cambridge, Mass.: Harvard East Asian Series.

Farquhar, Judith. 1994. *Knowing Practice: The Clinical Encounter of Chinese Medicine.* Boulder, Col.: Westview Press.

Fruehauf, Heiner. 1999. "Science, Politics, and the Making of 'TCM': Chinese Medicine in Crisis." *Journal of Chinese Medicine* 61: 1-17.

Hiller, S. M., and J. A. Jewell. 1983. *Health Care and Traditional Medicine in China, 1800-1982.* London: Routledge & Kegan Paul.

Horn, Joshua A. 1969. *Away with All Pests: An English Surgeon in People's China, 1954-1969.* New York: Monthly Review Press.

Hsu, Elisabeth. 1999. *The Transmission of Chinese Medicine.* Cambridge: Cambridge University Press.

Lampton, David L. 1977. *The Politics of Medicine in China: The Policy Process 1949-1977.* Folkstone: Dawson Publishing.

Lucas, AnElissa. 1982. *Chinese Medical Modernization: Comparative Policy Continuities, 1930s-1980s.* New York: Praeger.

Porkert, Manfred, Mark Howson, and Christian Ullmann. 1988. *Chinese Medicine: As a Scientific System, Its History, Philosophy and Practice, and How it Fits With the Medicine of the West.* New York: Morrow.

Porkert, Manfred. 1997. *Chinese Medicine Debased.* Dinkelscherben: Phainon.

Rosenthal, Marilyn M. 1987. *Health Care in the People's Republic of China: Moving Towards Modernization.* Boulder: Westview Press.

Scheid, Volker. 2002. *Chinese Medicine in Contemporary China: Plurality and Synthesis.* Durham, N.C.: Duke University Press.

Sidel, Victor W., and Ruth Sidel. 1973. *Serve the People: Observations on Medicine in the People's Republic of China.* Baltimore: Prot City Press.

Sivin, Nathan. 1988. *Traditional Medicine in Contemporary China.* Ann Arbor: University of Michigan, Center for Chinese Studies.

Chapter 10
Other East Asian Countries

In the course of their 2,000-year history, Chinese health and long life methods have also been transmitted into other East Asian countries, notably Vietnam, Korea, and Japan. In all three countries, they merged with local herbalism and shamanic practices, adapting to climate and flora, customs and mentality. As a result, they underwent specific local developments that created different perspectives and treatment variations.

The Chinese empire exerted a considerable political and cultural influence on its neighbors from an early time. Even in the Shang dynasty (1766-1122 B.C.E.), when turtle shell divination was at its height, trade routes extended all over the East Asian hemisphere. Under the Former Han (206-6 B.C.E.), Chinese military garrisons occupied areas as far west as modern Afghanistan and as far south as Vietnam; the Korean kingdoms were seen as vassal states with close connections to the Middle Kingdom; and Japan was known as a distant, somewhat strange land across the sea. The greatest imperial expansion in Chinese history occurred in the Tang dynasty (618-907), when numerous delegations went back and forth between countries.

The bulk of medical knowledge traveled to Vietnam, Korea, and Japan at this time. Only a few earlier events are known, including a delegation of Chinese physicians to Korea in 514, the translation of the *Pulse Classic* into Korean, the transmission of medical works to Japan by the Korean physician Te Lai and the Buddhist Zhi Cong, and a collection of acupuncture works transmitted to Japan in 552. In the early seventh century, a formal delegation of Japanese physicians reached China and the first classes in Chinese medicine in Japan were taught under imperial auspices by a Korean physician.

Texts continued to be transmitted and translated, so that by the mid-seventh century, the various documents associated with the *Yellow Emperor's Inner Classic, On Cold-Induced Disorders*, and the encyclopedic *Origins and Symptoms of Medical Disorders* (*Zhubing yuanhou lun*, dat. 610) were well known all over East Asia. Soon afterwards, Chinese medicine became the official health system of Heian Japan. In 733 another delegation of physicians came to China to study there for an entire decade, and in 753 the Chinese monk Jianzhen (Jap. Ganjin) arrived in Japan to transmit knowledge of medical treatments and herbs and to provide free medical services to the people. His work is honored today in a museum in the Shôsôin Temple in Nara; it includes also a collection of original ancient herbal remedies. Many of the active ingredients are still intact after thirteen centuries (see www.itmonline.org).

Not only spreading south and east, Chinese medicine around the same time also reached Tibet, whose king married a Chinese princess in 641. In her dowry, she brought books, instruments, and herbs, stimulating the translation of twenty-seven medical works and enhancing a general interest in medical matters which led to the invitation of physicians also from Persia and India. Tibetan medicine grew from these different strands. To the present day it uses diagnosis, pulses, and certain healing methods adopted from China.

The main event in this early phase of East Asian medical development is the Japanese compilation in 984 of the encyclopedic work *Essential Medical Methods* (*Ishinpô*, trl. Hsia et al. 1986), by the court physician Tamba no Yasuyori (912-995). Its thirty chapters mirror Tang medicine, citing passages from 204 ancient sources, most of them Chinese, in each case listing the causes and symptoms of diseases, then discussing healing therapies and longevity practices.

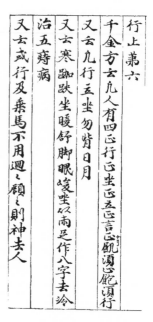

Following the Tang dynasty, China underwent a series of internal disputes and wars with Central Asian peoples, making easy contact and transmission of texts impossible. While connections resumed to a certain degree in the thirteenth century, the various East Asian countries increasingly began to develop their own systems and approaches.

Fig. 19. An excerpt from the *Essential Medical Methods*.

Thus, Vietnamese medicine developed into a two-part system: a northern medicine which closely imitated the Chinese model and a southern medicine which relied largely on locally grown herbs and family knowledge. Both are still active today, now contrasted with Western medicine (*thuoc tay*) and collectively called "our medicine" (*thuoc ta*). Northern medicine is essentially Chinese. Its concepts of *qi* (*khi*), yin-yang, the five phases, inner organs, and meridians, and its methods of diagnosis and treatment have become the mainstay of Vietnamese medical thinking. Within its overall framework, several uniquely Vietnamese concepts developed. One is that the heart is central—the emperor of the body and dwelling place of the spirit as well as a prime avenue for treatment. This is contrary to Chinese medicine, which uses a fluid model of understanding and whose physicians still hesitate to treat the heart directly (see www.vietnamwebsite.net; www.masean.org).

Another uniquely Vietnamese approach strongly emphasizes natural, environmental factors in the causation of disease and focuses on water and wind, not accidentally the same basic forces as in Chinese Fengshui. Vietnam is pervaded by waterways and relies heavily on irrigation for its rice agriculture. Like the country, so the body is seen as consisting of "governing palaces" and "storage depots," connected by "canals" or life-bringing arteries and meridians. Water as a basic of natural resources needs to flow in the right amount, subject to neither floods nor droughts. Similarly, wind is a key factor in Vietnam. Strong winds come from either north or south, bringing dryness and heat or cold, affecting the health and well-being of the individual. This emphasis, of course, also resonates with wind as a key pathogenic factor in ancient China, but in Vietnam it has pervaded the culture to a greater degree, linking wind with emotions, morals, and health (Craig, *Familiar Medicine*, 44-46).

Chinese medicine in Vietnam was codified variously. The most important work is the *Medical Recipes of the Lazy Man by the Sea* (*Hai Thuong y ton tam linh*), by Lan Ong (1720-1791). This vast encyclopedia of medical methods comprises sixty-six sections and includes discussions of pharmacology, pulse manipulation, pathologies, as well as special presentations on gynecology, obstetrics, pediatrics, hygiene, and physical exercises. Today it is taught in specialized departments of Western-oriented medical and pharmaceutical schools. This institutionalization is a fairly recent development. Traditionally physicians were trained in an apprenticeship system, following a specific master who would transmit his teaching orally rather than in an academic setting and through officially recognized textbooks. Not unlike a guru in a spiritual tradition, the master not only taught the student but was also responsible for giving him enough *qi* to face the rigors of practice.

This system of training has led to vast differences in quality and expertise among traditional Vietnamese doctors, causing an attitude of contempt for physicians and a sense of insecurity and apprehension. Unlike in other East Asian countries, where doctors came from all levels of society and were often treated with great respect and even honored by imperial favor, Vietnamese physicians were considered lowly members of society. Rather than being paid for their services, they received donations of food, clothing, and cash. These donations over time evolved into a *de facto* payment system, but the principle of low status and little pay remained intact and to the present day patients are expected not only to pay a given clinic's set fees but to hand a cash envelope to the physician in person. People who fail to pay the bribe are blacklisted and will not be seen by the doctor again (Craig, *Familiar Medicine*, 175).

It is thus not surprising that patients are leery of doctors and make their own decisions about treatments and drugs. Their first line of defense is a change in diet as influenced by southern, herbal medicine. If that does not work, a knowledgeable family member or neighbor may recommend a locally grown herbal remedy. From here, the patient consults a respected pharmacist and often starts to take antibiotics. Antibiotics are freely available over the counter and advertised widely. People use them with frightening nonchalance for various periods, but rarely for a full antibiotic cycle. When this fails and as a last resort, a doctor is consulted, and even then patients rely on local recommendations and get at least two opinions before again making up their own mind about what medicine to take when and in what quantities (Craig, *Familiar Medicine*, 65).

This system of patient-empowerment has stood the country in good stead during its independence since 1945 — a time characterized by civil war, the Vietnam War, Communism, and now Doi Moi or Renovation, the careful introduction of market principles and international opening. For much of this time, people had to rely on their own resources since medical services, run through the people's communes, were elementary at best. Most recently, the socialist health system has collapsed and people have to pay almost all medical expenses out of pocket, increasing their distrust and caution. Women are the key decision makers in this process, since they tend to inherit the local herbal lore and are in charge of the children. But men, too, eagerly discuss the merits and demerits of various pharmacists, doctors, and remedies (Craig, *Familiar Medicine*, 164-68). While this ensures a continued education of the people in medical matters and a great deal of self-awareness and medical thinking, which is for the most part still based on Chinese concepts, the disadvantage is that often treatments are haphazard and antibiotics are taken for no good cause nor in the properly prescribed manner, resulting in an increased antibiotic resistance, especially among children.

> **Exercise:** Reflect on the problem of patient empowerment in the light of the two extremes: the need for relying on ones' own resources due to lack of medical care and the control over medical decisions by an authorized individual or organization. Where do we stand on this scale in comparison to Vietnam? What is ideal?

In Korea, mainstream medicine was practiced by *hanuisa*, "Chinese medical practitioners" who coexisted successfully with indigenous shamanic healers and herbalists. It has brought forth four distinct independent developments. The first is the inclusion of Korean native plants in the East Asian pharmacopoeia, found in the *Sejong Pharmacopoeia* (*Sejong bonchohak*), ordered by King Sejong in 1493. This king is best known for his creation of *hangul*, the Korean phonetic alphabet. The compilation expanded the scope of Chinese herbal remedies, but did not alter the theoretical model of the system.

The second development is a unique emphasis on the five-phases model. In 1574, the Buddhist monk Sa'am expanded on the *Classic of Difficult Issues* by focusing on three chapters (68, 69, 75) that defined the associated phase points on each meridian, the "mother-child" relationship of meridians, as well as the controlling cycle. On this basis, he created the so-called Korean Four Point Constitutional method. It utilizes a specific pulse indication to diagnose imbalance in a given organ system, then provides a point prescription to allow practitioners to correct the imbalance. This uniquely Korean approach sets the trend for a strong focus on the five phases as the major theoretical model.

This approach was further expanded by the Korean scholar Hejun who, in 1603, was commanded by the king to record his knowledge of medicine. He composed the thirty-three volume work, *Treasured Reflections on Eastern Medicine* (*Dongui bogam*), covering techniques from acupuncture and moxibustion to physical manipulation, herbs, diets, and breathing techniques. Its underlying theoretical position again centers on the five phases, including even herbal components, thus breaking away from the Chinese model. The text also served a political dimension in its presentation of Korean medicine as a branch of Chinese practice and called it "Eastern Chinese" (*donghan*), contending that Korean practice was one aspect of Chinese medicine. This implied that Korea was one part of the greater Chinese cultural sphere and politically served as a justification for asking the Chinese to help against Japanese invasions.

The third distinct Korean development was the Four Constitutions method by Lee Jaema in 1894. A minor government official turned herbalist, he developed a theory that the body is born with an innate constitution which dictates the tendency for health or disease. By determining the patient's constitution, the practitioner can manage long-term care since he or she will be aware of likely disharmonies and diseases. The Four Constitutions are four body types, determined by the relationship of hip mass to ribcage mass, as well as the depth of the anterior superior iliac spine and the angle of the intercostals. They also involve specific physical sizes of the organs, a concept entirely new to East Asian medicine. Each constitutional type tends to have either a big organ which tends to be deficient (too large to be filled with *qi*) or a small organ which tends to be in excess (too small to hold all the *qi*). The Four Constitutions are:

> Greater Yang (*taeyang*): the person has a strong neck and slender waist; skilled at communicating, with talent for social acquaintances; large lungs, small liver.
>
> Lesser Yang (*soyang*): the person has a broad chest and small hips; has a warrior mentality and a talent for fulfilling appointed roles; large liver, small lungs.
>
> Greater Yin (*taeum*): the person has a thick waist and a weak neck; skilled at accomplishments, with a talent for home making and interior design; large kidneys, small spleen.
>
> Lesser Yin (*soum*): the person has broad hips and a weak chest; skilled at good conduct and a talent for good family relations; large spleen, small kidneys.

The heart as an organ is left out of the system since someone with a native heart constitution would enjoy a near perfect balance of the organs and be a sage. As for ordinary people, if a patient shows big-organ deficiency and small-organ excess, the prognosis for recovery is good and the treatment can be aggressive. If he or she shows big-organ excess and small-organ deficiency, the prognosis is poor and the treatment must be carefully administered to avoid iatrogenesis. The method, with numerous technical details, has been in use ever since its inception and in 1960 was expanded further by Kwon Dowon into the Eight Constitutions

Method, utilizing the binary yin-yang relationship and focusing more on acupuncture than on herbs.

The fourth and most recent innovation in Korean medicine is Korean Hand Acupuncture, developed by Yoo Taewoo in 1975. It recognizes fourteen meridians and 345 acupuncture points, all centered in the hands, which it treats in a variety of ways: small, thin needles, specially developed by Yoo; moxibustion for chronic diseases; T-Chim needles or "tacks" for extended therapy on acute problems; magnets held with a band-aid; electrical stimulation; emergency bleeding by pricking the finger tips; pressure through bump-covered stress-balls or rings; and general hand exercises.

Any of these methods can alleviate deficiencies, reduce excess, clear heat, and warm up cold. Using the hand is convenient and practical, and allows for a great deal of flexibility, as the same disease can be treated with different methods. The method is not invasive and does not need a major clinical setting; certain basic treatments can even be self-administered or given among friends. Common uses include smoking cessation, depression relief, fatigue recovery, and making children grow taller (see www.medcity.com/kom).

> **Exercise:** Take a toothpick, wooden match, or fingernail and press it on several spots in your hand. If you find an area that is sore, press or massage it.

Yoo's method became popular because he described it in *hangul* and in a non-technical style, since he and his students were not highly educated but practically minded. It spread around the world and, in 1980, was expanded by Park Jaewoo to include Hand and Foot Acupuncture. His method reorients the mapping system of the organs to the hands and also includes the feet as an avenue of treatment, involving also a five-phases treatment system based on the work of Sa'am.

Korean medicine today is alternative to allopathic treatments and often integrates Western biomedicine. Many patients receive both Western and Eastern treatments simultaneously (the so-called third medicine) and are examined by different doctors in a single appointment. They take Chinese herbs alongside Western pharmaceuticals and generally feel well taken care of. If they wished to consult with a purely Korean doctor, it would likely be an herbalist, since that is the only formally licensed branch of Korean medicine. Acupuncture, moxibustion, physical manipulation, and energy healing are still unregulated professions, whose practitioners acquire varying levels of skill through apprenticeships and by taking courses at small schools with no licensing or regulatory standards. One exception is the Modern School of Acupuncture in Seoul, whose director Lee Byoungkuk has distinguished himself as a major activist, pushing for a proper Korean acupuncture license.

Another area of conflict is the establishment of new government regulations that require all raw ingredients of traditional medicine, like herbs and animal parts, to be packaged and labeled, forcing many smaller shops out of business. The conception among practitioners is that while the government wishes to modernize their field, it is in fact preventing progress and innovation (see www.koreanmedicine.net).

Very similar tendencies also apply to the development of Chinese medicine in Japan, where several schools of medicine arose in the fifteenth century. The first is the School of Later Developments (Goseiha), founded by Tashiro Sanki (1465-1537) after an extended study period in China where he learned about the Earth Tonifying and Yin Moisturizing Schools of the Yuan dynasty. Following their lead, he developed a new understanding of how herbal medicines affected the organs and meridians, and he created a number of herbal combinations that have remained in active use ever since. Over the centuries the Goseiha school's practices have spread widely, further expanded by Manase Dôsan (1507-1594), the author of the *Textbook of Internal Medicine* (*Keitekishu*) and founder of a private medical school in Kyoto. He systematized the school's teachings further and added emphasis on the treatise *On Cold-Induced Disorders*, influencing it to the extent that it is sometimes called the Dôsan School.

Another major unique Japanese development is the School of Classical Formulas (Kohôha), which favored the continuation of old traditions and relied mainly on conformation theory. This involved matching the patient's symptomatic complexes to a particular ancient herbal or treatment formula, with no specific interpretation of where and how remedies worked within the meridian and organ system. The school's theoretical understanding, developed by Goto Gonzan (1659-1733), focused on the concept of qi-stagnation, which was seen as the main factor responsible for the development of diseases under adverse conditions, such as severe weather patterns or strong emotions. This was modified again by Todo Yoshimasu (1702-1773) who proposed that there was one basic toxin that entered the body and caused diseases, the differences in symptoms and illnesses being merely variations in toxin location. It could be diagnosed best through abdominal palpitation. Both theories are still current among Japanese practitioners (see www.itmonline.org).

In acupuncture, a major school was the Nondivision School (Mubunha) which, like the Korean trend started by Sa'am, followed the *Classic of Difficult Issues* but also used the detailed abdominal palpitation proposed by the School of Classical Formulas. Popular to the present day, it uses a diagnostic system based on identifying deficient and excess *qi* conditions within the meridians. Beyond this, the Japanese developed fine-gauge needles for the performance of very shallow needling, especially applied by blind practitioners who became increasingly expert at acupuncture and massage. This, in turn, led to the creation of the first guide-tube for needle insertions by Sugiyama Waiichi in the late 1600s. Both shallow insertions and the guide-tube are hallmarks of Japanese acupuncture.

As in China, Western medicine was introduced by missionaries and traders in the sixteenth century and was acknowledged as a possible alternative to traditional methods. It rose to the fore when modernization and westernization began in the Meiji period (1868-1902) and education in Chinese medicine was almost given up completely. Acupuncture was divorced from traditional theory and reinterpreted in a Western medical model, considered to work through nervous system stimulation. This resulted in a drastic reduction in efficacy to the point where acupuncture was rejected as useless and superstitious by the Japanese medical establishment. Opinions changed gradually in the 1920s, and an attempt was undertaken to rediscover lost medical arts. Books touted their miraculous healing effects, and a flurry of interest in old methods arose.

In the acupuncture community, the work of Yanagiya Sôrei is of particular importance. He used and publicized the *Classic of Difficult Issues* and five-phases methods of Sa'am, describing them as indigenous Japanese medicine. They became the foundation of Japanese acupuncture as it is still practiced today — officially licensed but separate from herbal medicine. Acupuncturists receive licenses after three years in vocational college, while herbal training programs are attached to pharmacy colleges and licensure in Western pharmacology is required for attendance.

Exercise: How are complementary medical methods taught and licensed in your country? What, in your opinion, is the best way for their organization? Should acupuncturists and herbalists be trained like allopathic doctors? How much Western training should they have?

In addition to the separation of acupuncture and herbal treatments, there is little effort in Japan to integrate Western and Eastern medicine into one system but patients choose one or the other. Both are equally covered by national health insurance, which reimburses two thirds of most medical expenses. On the other hand, allopathic practitioners are well aware of traditional herbs, and 72 percent prescribe them in one form or the other.

While, therefore, traditional medicine has been largely integrated into the medical systems of China, Korea, and Vietnam, they remain separate both in Japan and Western countries. Even there, however, a growing portion of the population has come to appreciate Chinese medical methods for their efficacy and non-intrusive nature. In Europe and the U.S. about 75 percent of the population has made use of complementary methods, and the numbers are increasing. More and more studies show the efficacy of acupuncture in relieving pain and nausea and helping with drug addictions and chronic conditions. Developed along various independent lines in other East Asian countries, Chinese medicine today is unfolding to further dimensions in its newest setting, the West.

Further Readings

Craig, David. 2002. *Familiar Medicine: Everyday Health Knowledge and Practice in Today's Vietnam*. Honolulu: University of Hawai'i Press.

Finckh, Elisabeth. 1988. *Studies in Tibetan Medicine*. Ithaca: Snow Lion Publications.

Ho, P. Y., and F. P. Lisowski. 2000. *A Brief History of Chinese Medicine and Its Influence*. River Edge, NJ: World Scientific Publishing.

Hsia, Emil C. H., Ilza Veith, and Robert H. Geertsma, trans. 1986. *The Essentials of Medicine in Ancient China and Japan: Yasuyori Tamba's Ishinpô*. 2 vols. Leiden: E. Brill.

Kelder, Peter. 1975. *Tibetan Secrets of Health and Vitality*. Wellingborough: The Aquarian Press.

Nakayama, Shigeru. 1984. *Academic and Scientific Traditions in China, Japan, and the West*. Tokyo: Tokyo University Press.

Rister, Robert. 1999. *Japanese Herbal Medicine: The Healing Art of Kampo*. Garden City Park, NY: Avery Publishing Group.

Chapter 11

Acupuncture in America

Acupuncture was first practiced in the U.S. by Chinese immigrants in the nineteenth century, especially on the West Coast. It became known to the wider American public in 1971, when President Richard Nixon visited China to begin diplomatic relations. During the visit James Reston, a writer for the *Washington Post*, came down with an infected appendix and had to undergo surgery in Beijing. Offered acupuncture for anesthesia and post-surgical pain, he was very impressed with its effects.

Since then acupuncture has become quite common. Although it was outlawed together with all forms of complementary medicine in various states—as, for example, in Illinois from 1983 to 1993—making its practice a felony of the same caliber as rape and assault, by 1995 most states had regulatory laws and practice standards as well as licensing procedures. Special acupuncture schools were founded, and today the typical career of an acupuncturist begins with a four-year training program, which includes basic courses in biomedical knowledge as well as training in Chinese worldview, *qi*-theory, needling techniques, moxibustion, herbs, Qigong, and other methods of *qi*-balancing.

Exercise: Go to the web and look up the acupuncture school nearest you. What is their program? How is it organized? How much does it cost?

Acupuncture schools require a college degree and bestow a certificate, then arrange for successful students to take the state licensing examination. They are not yet on equal par with medical schools, whether allopathic (M.D.) or naturopathic (N.D.), but there is trend in this direction. Similarly there is a growing tendency for insurance companies to cover acupuncture and other complementary treatments. If paid privately, a treatment costs between $50.00 and $100.00 (www.aomalliance.org; www.aaom. org).

Acupuncture in the U.S. is practiced in all its varieties. The mainland Chinese version (TCM) is most common, but there are also practitioners that follow Korean, Japanese, Vietnamese, and even European schools. Techniques are manifold. There is acupuncture with stainless-steel nee-

117

dles and with medicinal needles that inject specific herbs, medication, or vitamins into acupuncture points. There are also electro-acupuncture, which involves small electric impulses being inserted through the needles; auriculotherapy or ear acupuncture which focuses on needles placed on specific points in the ears; and laser acupuncture where laser beams are directly applied to the points, making the use of needles superfluous (www.americanacupuncture.com; www.acupuncturetoday.com).

Acupuncture in the U.S. is widespread but not universally accepted. The medical community tends to accept healing methods only if and when they have been proven with their own tests, preferably in double-blind studies. Since the existence of *qi* is still a sore point among natural scientists, its manipulation with needles or burning herbs is not a favored approach to diseases. Although there is no scientific understanding of how acupuncture works, a few theories have come forward. One says that acupuncture works because it goes to the "gate" of the pain, which does not come from a single nerve root but involves the entire central nervous system. The stimulation from the needles jams the lower nerve bundles and the pain signals cannot get through. Another theory involves endorphins, i.e., opiates in the brain that control pain perception. According to this, the needles stimulate the release of these opiates, creating a natural form of anesthesia while also enhancing the functioning of other glands, such as the thyroid and pituitary which regulate body hormones.

A third theory on the workings of acupuncture relies on local zones or dermatomes. It says that the body has reference zones for the various inner organs which coincide with the segmental distribution of somatic sensory nerve-fibers. These fibers enter the spinal cord at the same level as the fibers coming from the related organ, so that, for example, the heart is connected to the chest, shoulder, and arm. The needles in acupuncture trigger a reaction across the dermatomes to influence the working of the inner organs. Yet another theory focuses on heterostasis. It claims that acupuncture as such has no healing properties whatsoever but stimulates the body to produce more of its own natural balancing agents, such as hormones. Doing so, it improves the immune reaction and leads to healing, not only on the surface but at the root of the problem, and increases overall balance and health. Pain is relieved because as one allows the body to release good energy, one feels better overall (Filshie and White, *Medical Acupuncture*).

In addition to these theories, many scientific studies have been undertaken. However, as documented variously in *The Clinical Journal of Pain* and other journals, the tendency in Western experiments is to ignore the traditional parameters of Chinese healing, such as the five phases, *qi*, and blood, and replace individually tailored treatments with randomized, double-blind, and placebo-controlled trials. Acupuncture therapy is reduced to a mathematical formula of acupuncture points, and all patients receive the same treatment. When differentiated treatments are applied, the numbers tend to be too small to be statistically significant.

A big problem is the sham effect. As the "NIH Consensus on Acupuncture" of 1997 states, "Placement of a needle in any position elicits a biological response that complicates the interpretation of studies involving sham acupuncture." Some studies have tried to solve this problem using a "sham-laser," which emits a red light but no beam. Still, this does not address the placebo or sham effect properly, and it is not surprising that statistical analysis has shown that the difference between the sham and verum groups is typically not significant—actual acupuncture not being based on a proper diagnosis and thus not very efficient either.

Besides clinical trials, anecdotal and systematic evidence from acupuncturists has created an impressive body of knowledge on the workings of acupuncture. The NIH panel on acupuncture reviewed both scientific studies and other evidence and concluded that there was strong evidence that it helps with post-operative and chemotherapy nausea and pain; good evidence that it helps with other pain, such as menstrual cramps, tennis elbow, and fibromyalgia; some evidence that it relieves addiction, stroke, carpal-tunnel syndrome, osteoarthritis, and headaches; and rather little evidence that it helps people to quit smoking.

Acupuncture is generally recognized in the U.S. as acceptable for anesthesia, analgesia, allergies, circulatory disorders, dermatological conditions, intestinal disorders (colitis, hiccups, constipation), musculoskeletal disorders (arthritis, tendonitis, bursitis), genital disorders, respiratory disorders (cold, cough, bronchitis), and some psychiatric problems (insomnia, fatigue, depression, anxiety, neuroses, addictions). It has also been conclusively shown that when used immediately after a trauma or shock, acupuncture can reduce blood pressure and alleviate the overall condition of the patient, thereby eliminating the need for drugs and ensuring a greater survival rate. (see http://acupuncture.8k.com; www.who.int/medicines)

When applied in anesthesia, patients are pain free but not unconscious. Its application in the operating room evolved in modern China after post-operative pain had been reduced significantly with needles. In the early stages, as many as a hundred needles were inserted before an operation. Later, techniques were refined, the number of needles was greatly reduced, and physicians learned how it felt when the *qi* arrived in the proper spot. It was also found that needles had to be rotated periodically for the analgesic effect to continue and to prevent the patient from experiencing pain, a problem that was greatly alleviated through the use of electrical acupuncture.

Acupuncture anesthesia is not for everyone. It can be quite unsettling to be conscious of the activities in the operating room and to listen to the surgeons' dialogue. If selected, however, the likelihood is that the procedure is safe and without side-effects. It is especially useful for surgery on the head, neck, arms, and legs, as well as in procedures that last less than two hours. While applied in China without other measures, in the West it tends to be administered in combination with biomedical drugs. Even then, acupuncture analgesia is less expensive, lessens the impact on the respiratory, digestive, and other systems of the body, and ensures a faster recovery (Chai-hsi, *Acupuncture Anesthesia*).

Exercise: Would you consider acupuncture anesthesia for a major surgical procedure? Would you recommend it to a family member? If so, why and under what circumstances? If not, what are your hesitations?

Another popular use of acupuncture in the U.S. is for drug addiction. As such it has been used in Hong Kong since 1972 when an opium addict, ready to undergo neurosurgery, had acupuncture anesthesia. Needles with an electric charge were inserted at hand, arm and ear points. After a short time, the man found that his withdrawal symptoms were gone; he continued acupuncture treatments, never had the surgery, and has remained drug free. Since 1974, similar treatments have also been available in the U.S. They usually involve the placement of tiny needles in each ear at points related to the major organs, releasing endorphins that reduce drug cravings, ease withdrawal symptoms, and increase relaxation (www.acupuncture.com/faq-all.htm#2).

The therapy works best if treatments are received daily for the first two weeks and then gradually lessened. If relapses occur or something stressful in the patient's life happens, additional treatments should be given. However, even if followed faithfully, the physical treatments alone tend to be insufficient, and social and personal changes are necessary. Successful quitters typically are also involved in other forms of rehabilitation, such as the twelve-step programs offered through Alcoholics Anonymous or Narcotics Anonymous.

A major case study was undertaken in 1989 in Dade County, Florida, and according to its 1995 report, of 6,000 drug addicts rehabilitated with acupuncture, 3,480 were successful and are substance-free, while 1,200 remained enrolled in the treatment. Normally 60% of people arrested on drug charges are rearrested; here the re-arrest rate was under 40% (Mitchell, *Fighting Drug Abuse*). Since then, other Florida counties have adopted the treatment, making it an alternative to jail time. It has spread to various states, gradually creating a new culture of drug rehabilitation.

Another widespread problem in American society is the prevalence of headaches and migraines, a form of intense and often chronic head pain that can be piercing, throbbing, or pulsing. Unlike plain head aches, migraines tend to come with other debilitating symptoms, such as nausea and vomiting as well as sensitivity to light, sound, and movement, which cause more disruption in the sufferer's daily life. 11 percent of Americans suffer from migraines, untold numbers have tension headaches. As documented in the journal *Headache*, Western medicine tends to use pharmaceuticals and pain-killers for treatment. These are effective in about 70% of cases but tend to treat mainly the surface symptoms and ignore deeper energetic and lifestyle imbalances.

Acupuncture, too, can be used superficially, needling points at the back of the neck for immediate relief. However, the tendency here is to go to the root of the problem, seen as a larger pattern of wayward *qi*, which is different in every individual. Treating this and addressing wider issues of lifestyle, guiding patients to get regular sleep, meals, and exercise, acupuncture is able not only to reduce the frequency and severity of attacks, but even eliminate them completely. It provides a safe, individualized alternative to pharmacological treatments, with minimal risk and the potential for clearing up deep, ingrained patterns of disharmony. Again, acupuncture therapy, as Mark Seem points out, is perceived less as a direct, objective treatment of dysfunction than a prod to the body-mind to remember how to restore appropriate functioning and to heal itself (*Acupuncture Imaging*, 47).

From an acupuncture point of view, headaches as well as many other common ailments in American society are caused by a lifestyle of stress, shallow breathing, and fast food. Subjecting the body to these factors results in a permanent constriction of the adrenals and the upper chest and back muscles, which in turn leads to agitated emotional states, inappropriate anger, constriction in the stomach and diaphragm, as well as in the chest and throat areas. All these in the Chinese system are symptoms of constricted liver *qi*. If not treated in time, this constriction will impact the middle heater and the Penetrating Vessel, causing an even stronger disruption between the upper and lower regions in the body. The symptoms associated with this energetic condition are stomach ulcers, acid reflux, chronic fatigue syndrome, and immune deficiency disorders that may open the doors to viruses and potentially can result in AIDS (Seem, *Acupuncture Imaging*). For all of them, acupuncture offers a first release of the energetic imbalance that can then be followed by appropriate changes in lifestyle and breathing patterns.

Thus even in cases of AIDS, acupuncture, herbs, diet, and Qigong are applied. As the energetic disruption at this stage is already far advanced, none of these will cure the disease, but they can help to alleviate symptoms and the side effects of Western medications. AIDS in Chinese medicine tends to be defined as a form of toxic heat that invades first the liver, spleen, and stomach, then moves on to other inner organs, gradually consuming the entire body.

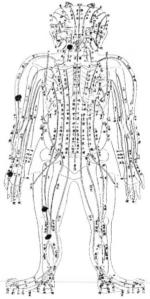

Treatments match this diagnosis, emphasizing St-36 and Sp-4 to tonify the stomach and spleen meridians, and reducing toxic heat with the help of LI-4, LI-11, Sp-10, and Bl-40 in the mid-back (Zheng and Hsu, *AIDS*). Treatments have to be taken regularly and are intensified as the disease progresses. A key figure in this pioneering treatment is Mary Kay Ryan in Chicago (www.qigongalliance.com).

Acupuncture and Chinese herbs are also used in cases of Attention Deficit Disorder (ADD) and Attention Deficit Hyperactivity Disorder (ADHD), a hyperkinetic syndrome that affects the brain and nervous system. Its origins are a matter of debate, and no single cause has been identified. The leading school of thought points to heredity, although others blame deficiencies in amino acids, high artificial sugar intake,

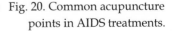

Fig. 20. Common acupuncture points in AIDS treatments.

and other diet issues. There are also those who believe that ADD does not exist at all, but diagnosis and treatment are an attempt at classroom standardization and behavioral molding. The most common treatment in the West is a drug known as Ritalin, a mild amphetamine which has a calming effect on the nervous system and is effective in 70 percent of cases. Dietary solutions with decreased intake of sugar, preservatives, and caffeine, along with taking supplements of iron, magnesium, and zinc are also effective about 50 percent of the time.

In Chinese medicine, ADD and ADHD are seen as a form of yin deficiency. This can be due to hereditary causes or to depletion through synthetic foods or other weaknesses. It often shows up dominantly in the kidney meridian, the prime carrier of yin and *jing* in the body and the root of marrow and brain tissue, but it may also affect the liver channel. Alternatively, the patient may suffer from phlegm obstruction of the heart, which leads to an inability to concentrate and general confusion.

Diagnosis differs according to the individual presented, and so do the remedies. Herbs prescribed nourish yin, dissolve phlegm, pacify spirit, and subdue yang. In comparative tests, they had better results than the 70 percent effectiveness of Ritalin. Acupuncture is also used to tonify the yin meridians and release excessive yang. Common treatment points are Lv-2 and Lv-3 to sooth agitated yang, Lu-11 for confusion, GV-24 for restlessness, PC-7 for lack of concentration, and Bl-15, the heart point of the bladder meridian in the upper back, for hyperactivity.

> **Exercise:** Go to the web and look up other predominant areas in which acupuncture is applied today. Where, in your opinion, can acupuncture have a greater impact in the future? Should it be better integrated? Should it be studied more?

Another growing branch of U.S. acupuncture is in veterinary practice where it is often used with biomedical treatments. It is one branch of AVM or Alternative Veterinary Medicine, defined as "diagnostic and treatment modalities or systems of medicine not commonly taught in veterinary medical schools" (www.altvetmed.com). Like Chinese medicine, AVM views the patient in holistic terms, taking into account the entire animal and its surroundings and not just immediate symptoms. It has a strong focus on prevention, correcting and enhancing functions in animals that may seem normal to biomedically trained practitioners (e.g., hairballs for cats or red-line gums in dogs), and strives to provide a fulfilling lifestyle to its patients, making sure their nutrition is well balanced, they get enough exercise, and they are emotionally satisfied. Unlike acupuncture for humans, alternative treatments for pets have been recognized officially. In 1996, the American Veterinary Medical Association stated that sufficient clinical and anecdotal evidence exists to suggest real benefits from a number of unconventional approaches, thus giving its seal of approval to the practice (see www.avma.org).

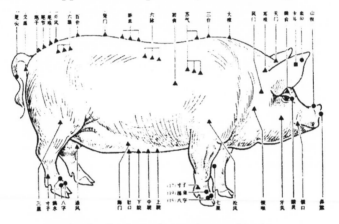

Fig. 21. Traditional acupoints on the pig.

To date about 400 veterinarians are also certified acupuncturists. They work predominantly on horses, dogs, and cats; to a lesser degree on dolphins, turtles, and others. Diagnosis follows the same four examinations as for human beings. It begins with looking at the coat, eyes, nose, ears, walking style, and overall behavior as well as the tongue, each of which may reveal an untoward pattern. Palpitation or touching may find sore spots in specific areas, symptomatic in the meridian network and thus indicative of some deeper internal problem. Hearing involves listening to the bark or meow, and inquiring whether the animal has had a change in common patterns. To get a better understanding of the individual's nature, the patient is also characterized in terms of the five phases. A "metal" cat, for example has "healthy, slow, and fluid movements . . . reflecting the quality of autumn light . . . and is soft, loving, quiet, and serious" (Zidonis and Snow, *Acu-Cat*, 30). Because metal is associated with the lungs, such a cat tends towards respiratory and immune-system problems. There is comparatively little asking of the animal directly, but its owner can usually relate the relevant problems.

Once diagnosis is established, treatment techniques include plain needling, electric needling, bloodletting, heat, massage, and low-power lasers. Acupuncture points are identified in one of two ways: either by transposing points taken from human beings onto the animal body, or by going back to the traditional Chinese model, which has centuries of records on animal acupuncture. The transpositional model is easier for human-trained acupuncturists but has the disadvantage that important points in people are hard to match in animals. The traditionalist model is more reliable but harder to access since not much of the literature has been translated. Also, most texts in traditional China deal with domestic animals such as horses, cows, sheep, and pigs, and leave out any mention of cats and dogs, the preferred patients of today. The tendency is to use a mixture of models and rely on the growing literature of contemporary experience.

Exercise: Go to the following links and learn more about animal acupuncture and its application. What strikes you in particular? Links include: www.cah.com; www.aava.org; www.acupuncturetoday.com; www.lid.com; www.catdoctor.com; www.animal-health-directory.com.

Unlike some more invasive biomedical procedures, acupuncture treatments do not hurt. Especially small needles used in household pets are entirely painless. Some larger needles used for horses and larger animals may cause some discomfort as they pass through the skin, but they too are painless once in place. Accordingly, animals tend to be friendly toward needles and usually sleep peacefully during treatment. This alone is a great advantage. Another benefit is that there is less potential for infection and that the treatment is less time consuming. Acupuncture for animals has been found very effective for pain control and also as a supplement to other treatments for a variety of disorders, such as respiratory, gastrointestinal, neurological, musculoskeletal, reproductive, dermatological, and urinary problems. The cost is comparatively high. A short session of three to five minutes may cost about $50.00 (www.ivas.org). For example:

> A 9-year old Pekinese named Noel was reluctant to walk, acting painful, unhappy, and lethargic. She was presented to her regular veterinarian because she was not "acting like her normal self." Blood tests came back normal and the owner was told that nothing was wrong and not to worry. However, over the next several months Noel's attitude continued to deteriorate as well as her general physical condition and activity. X-rays were taken, yet results were again inconclusive.
>
> When presented to a veterinary acupuncturist, Noel was diagnosed as having *qi* blockage and blood stagnation in the bladder meridian. An acupuncture treatment was done.

One week later Noel returned for re-evaluation and was walking normally. She was happy and reported to be back to her normal bossy behavior in the household.

A black cocker spaniel named Sable came to the acupuncturist after a lifelong history of allergy problems. Allergy testing had shown positive to all environmental allergens. She had a dull hair coat, multiple pustules all over her body, and chronic ear infection. She had been treated with steroids and multiple antibiotics for most of her life. Acupuncture was started on a weekly basis. Chinese herbs and dietary supplements were also implemented.

Sable was slow to respond, and it was almost two months before significant change could be noted. The ear problems disappeared, the hair coat grew to be shiny and full, and the itching stopped. She is now happy, active, and is seen every 2-3 months for a "tune-up" treatment. She is no longer taking any drugs for her condition, but continues to maintain a healthy lifestyle with herbal supplements and periodic acupuncture treatments. (www.apvet.com)

Further Readings

Altman, Sheldon. 1995. *Acupuncture for Animals*. New York: Chaus Corporation.

Chai-hsi E.L., ed. 1976. *Getting to Know Acupuncture Anesthesia*. Philadelphia: Dorrance & Company.

Filshie J. and White A., eds. 1998. *Medical Acupuncture: A Western Scientific Approach*. New York: Churchill Livingstone.

Goldstein, Martin. 1999. *The Nature of Animal Healing*. New York: Ballantine.

Mitchell, Ellinor R. 1995. *Fighting Drug Abuse with Acupuncture: The Treatment That Works*. Berkeley: Pacific View Press.

NIH, ed. 1997. *NIH Consensus Development Conference on Acupuncture*. Bethesda: NIH.

Seem, Mark D. 1990. *Acupuncture Imaging: Perceiving the Energy Pathways of the Body*. New York: Inner Traditions.

Zhang, Qingcai, and Hong-Yen Hsu 1995. *AIDS and Chinese Medicine*. Long Beach, Calif.: Oriental Healing Arts Institute.

Zidonis, Nancy A. and Amy. Snow. 1998. *Acu-Cat: A Guide to Feline Acupressure*. Denver, Col.: Tallgrass Publishers.

Chapter 12
Fengshui

Besides treatment by a trained physician or therapist, the Chinese health system also provides a number of methods for individuals to control the flow of *qi* in their interaction with the environment, foodstuffs, and other people, thus creating health and harmony for themselves. Most importantly, people should be conscious about where they live and how they arrange their homes, because the *qi* in one's immediate physical environment is a key contributor to the way one feels. The practice of placing oneself most auspiciously into the physical setting is called Fengshui, a term which literally means "wind and water" and is also known as "geomancy." Over the past decade, this has become popular in the West, where it is used to provide ways for the most harmonious *qi*-flow and thus the best possible fortune through the siting of houses and furniture.

Fengshui goes back far in Chinese history and has always been part of the larger medical enterprise. As Gary Seaman notes, Fengshui is as much medicine as acupuncture in that both depend on a doctrine of macrocosm-microcosm correspondence and seek to channel or alter natural processes for purposes of curing sickness and securing general well-being ("Winds, Waters," 75-76). This, moreover, is found also in other traditional cultures, such as the Indian Vastu, and more recently can be related to the Gaia theory, the notion of the earth as a living entity. A theory first advanced in the 1970s by James Lovelock, it maintains that the earth has consciousness and that the planet as a whole participates actively in its shaping and exchanges energies with all beings living on its surface — rejoicing in certain activities and deploring others.

The Gaia theory notes that the earth has a tendency to optimize conditions for terrestrial life. In a history of 4.5 aeons or 1,000 million years, it should statistically have developed climatic changes toward extreme temperatures. However, this never happened. The earth always kept things temperate, which shows that it tends to optimize the varying conditions by developing new agents that produce gases or chemicals counteracting problematic situations. Thus Gaia as the living earth can be understood as the sum total of different individual modifications in planetary development, as the total interconnected network of all species. This is, moreover, an ongoing thing. The earth continues to adapt and modify in accordance with various developments and to match its patterns to the network of species.

Gaia, like other living organisms, has vital organs at its core and redundant organs on its periphery. It is thus much easier for the earth to alter things on its outside but it resists changes in things deep inside. For example, during the ice age all above and below 45 degrees latitude froze over, which was about thirty percent of the earth's surface. Even with this amount of freezing, the planet still functioned, since its core in the center remained untouched. It is therefore less dangerous to alter climates and physical conditions in the far north or south of the planet and more hazardous to modify things around the equator. The cutting down of the rain forests is likely to have a greater impact on global conditions that any changes affected around the poles.

The scientific understanding of the living earth closely matches the Fengshui vision of ancient China. The earth is alive and in many ways is analogous to the human body. Any activity that interferes with it impacts on the health and fortune of the people. Rivers and hills are an integrated system and are often described in terms of yin and yang animals, tigers and dragons. Within the earth, moreover, there are qi-flow arteries which, like the ley lines described in England, crisscross the earth. Like the blood vessels in the human body they transport vital qi and have to be open and clear for the organism to be healthy. One should thus always build in close alliance with these arteries and not interrupt them because that would cause qi stagnation and obstruction in the planet. Houses and cemeteries are accordingly placed in an exact configuration with the patterns of nature, taking into account the directions, lighting, natural contours, and overall energetic structure of the space in question.

Historically Fengshui began as the siting of graves, as part of the belief that ancestral spirits could only rest properly and benefit the living if their bodies, the manifestation of the material soul, was placed in harmony with the earth. Also, the essence of the buried skeleton was thought to exert an influence on living relatives, not unlike the resonance between light waves or sounds. The grave was thus a place of transformation for the dead and a source of vitality for the living (Seaman, "Winds, Waters," 87-88). Since, moreover, the dead were considered yin and the living yang, graves were sited in shady spots, on the northern side of hills and in valleys. The exact direction and layout of the grave had to match the birth and death dates of the person in question, creating a direct and inescapable influence on the good fortune for the surviving family. Even Daoists and Buddhists who left their families to become recluses paid close attention to the practice, since they believed that they could only attain higher stages of spirituality and immortality if their dead relatives were at peace in the otherworld. As a result, medieval Daoists not only performed elaborate rituals for the salvation and transfer of the ancestors to the realm of immortals, but also concerned themselves with the correct placement of their earthly resting places.

Exercise: Reflect on the role of the dead in our lives. How do you feel about family continuity, graves, and the presence of death? Has our culture gained or lost in comparison with ancient China?

Fengshui was taken very seriously in traditional China. An early record notes that the general Meng Tian, the builder of the first Great Wall around 220 B.C.E. committed suicide for having violated the dragon arteries of the earth. Another story tells how the official Guo Pu (276-324 C.E.) selected a site for his mother's grave by finding the course of the earth's living *qi*. He placed it one hundred paces from a river and thereby created great good fortune for himself and his family. He later became known as a major practitioner of Fengshui and his name appears linked with various Fengshui books, such as the well-known *Grave Classic (Zangjing)*. His biography is also the first work to use the term *fengshui*; before then the practice was called the analysis of *kanyu*, which literally means "cover and support," symbols of heaven and earth.

Going beyond the siting of graves, Fengshui principles were also applied to residences for the living. In the early stages, the dominant method was to determine the correct position of one's doorway in relation to the five phases. This method was not called Fengshui either, but known as the "art of planning residences" (*tuzhai shu*). Later, the concern shifted from the placement of the front door to the complex relationship of the building to the formations of the surrounding hills, valleys, and streams. People began to see their lives as influenced by the *qi* of the wind (*feng*) from the hills and the water (*shui*) from the streams, and they felt the urge to establish themselves in as much harmony with these forces as possible.

Fengshui today is practiced in four major schools: the Form School, the Compass School, the Intuitive School, and the Tantric School. The Form School is the oldest; it uses the shape of the landscape and other buildings to determine the patterns of the home. The Compass School also goes back far in history; it uses the diviner's compass and applies cosmological data, such as people's birth dates, directions, and solar and lunar stations to determine the greatest auspiciousness. Combining divination, religion, and astrology, it is the most complicated form of Fengshui and is not practiced by laymen. The Intuitive School is a more modern development which also involves a professional: a Fengshui practitioner closely in tune with *qi*-flow patterns comes to one's home and feels what needs to be done. Another modern school is the Tantric School, presented by the Black Sect of Tantric Buddhism. It relies on the identification of eight corners inside the house or room to enhance good fortune (www.fastfengshui.com; www.qi-whiz.com; www.wofs.com).

All schools focus on the basic analysis of two major forms of *qi*, analogous to the medical diagnosis of excess and deficiency. They are *shaqi* and *siqi*. *Shaqi*, literally "killing *qi*," is fast moving or rushing *qi*. It moves along straight lines and is found in pointed arrows and angular forms. Moving very fast, it takes away health and good fortune. An example is the placement of a house at the top of a T-junction. The *qi* from the road rushes straight at it and through it, taking positive energies away with it. But even ordinary entrances to a house or compound are in danger and should be protected. As a result, in traditional China the main entrance to a compound is usually blocked off to the street by the so-called spirit wall: a free-standing wall slightly broader than the gateway that is set inside the main wall right after the gate.

Other common locations of *shaqi* include staircases that rise straight up from the front door of the house, long corridors, and a window directly across from the door of a room. In all cases, these long, straight, pathways invite the *qi* to rush through, taking good fortune with it. It can be slowed down and mellowed with the help of a screen, plant, or curtain. Then there are the sink and toilet, where water flows out of the house, another drain of *qi*. In traditional China, bath houses and outhouses were completely separate from the dwelling and placed in their own Fengshui environment. In our apartments today, the bathroom should be between other rooms and the lid of the toilet should be kept closed. It is also important to avoid placing key items, such as the stove, bed, or desk in a *shaqi* location.

The other major form of *qi* is *siqi*, literally "dead *qi*." Blocked *qi* or obstructed *qi*, it is deficient because it cannot move freely. *Siqi* is found in all types of clutter--whether unused items or an overabundance of appreciated possessions, such as too many plants, books, dishes, clothes, and the like. Fengshui clutter does not have to be in the house itself; even piles disregarded stuff stored in other locations can have a negative impact. In other words, any assembly of material objects that does not let *qi* pass through freely is detrimental to one's well-being and should be cleaned out. Another form of blocked *qi* appears in dirty windows, dark corners of the house, and various heavy areas and objects. Cleaning helps, as does the creation of more light through the placement of lamps or mirrors. In addition, pathways of *qi* may be obstructed—doors that do not open all the way, blocked drain pipes, and the like. Again, it is important to keep things clear and open.

The ideal form of *qi* flow in and around one's residence is one of balance. There should be nice rounded shapes, open corners, a pleasant atmosphere, and ideally the presence of all colors of the five phases and the various aspects of yin and yang (heavy and light, dark and bright, soft and hard). When all aspects are represented in every room, *qi* can flow harmoniously, and one will find health and good fortune.

Within this framework, the Form School focuses on the placement of the house. Ideally there should be rich vegetation and some wildlife, showing that the ground is fertile and the *qi* is prosperous; barren hills and deserts should be avoided. In terms of the social environment, it is good to be near parks, gardens, playgrounds, spiritual centers, health areas, and schools—locations of vibrant *qi*. It is advisable to avoid hospitals, cemeteries, power stations, prisons, butcheries, and industrial estates.

Also, the house should be protected by nature, i.e., be located on the slope of a hill or near a higher building. It is detrimental to be on top of a hill or a cliff, since that creates exposure and invites rushing *qi*. Nor should one live underneath a cliff or in the shadow of a very high building, because this creates oppression and limitation. The landscape, moreover, should reflect all five phases—pointy (fire), tall (wood), angular (metal), undulating (water), and round (earth). It is also helpful to examine the shape of the landscape in terms of animal forms. Here the optimal shape is that resembling a dragon, while hills looking like tigers or rabbits are less auspicious.

In addition, the house should be well lighted and exposed to plenty of sun. Ideally it should face south and not be located along the northern slopes of hills or in other cool, shady areas. Having a body of water or an undulating road nearby is helpful, since water brings fertility and roads create good flowing *qi*. But again there can be too much of a good thing, and closeness to the ocean and/or a busy highway should be avoided. Also, the earth arteries or dragon veins need to be examined by a Feng-shui master, since they are invisible to normal eyes. As much as possible, the house and its nearby roads should not disrupt their flow but be in alignment with them. If they are cut off, wealth and happiness will drain away—a feature feared when the first railroads were built in China, leading to massive protests.

The Compass School deals both with the siting of houses and interior structures. It uses the diviner's compass or "cosmic board" (*luopan*), a multilevel model of the universe that consists of a square bottom plate representing earth and is divided according to the eight directions. On top of this is a round, movable plate representing heaven that is inscribed with characters signifying the days of the sixty-day cycle, the twenty-eight lunar mansions, and the twenty-four solar stations of the year (Harper, "Han Cosmic Board").

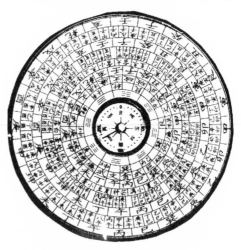

Fig. 22. The diviner's compass or cosmic board.

An example for the workings of the Compass School is the identification of a fate number based on an individual's year of birth which then determines certain auspicious and inauspicious directions. For example, if you were born in 1983, your fate number would be seven and your auspicious directions would be southwest (for health), west (overall harmony), northwest (wealth), and northeast (relationships), the other directions being inauspicious. To get the best fortune according to this method, the main door of the house and your bedroom should be in one of the auspicious directions, while the bathroom could be in a less fortunate place. Also, it would not be too problematic if a section of the house in one of your inauspicious directions were missing altogether. The system gets more complicated if you have more than one person in the house and their fate numbers do not overlap. In that case, a decision based on seniority or importance in the family can be made, using the dominant person's Fengshui to arrange the house; or again, the family could decide which issues to concentrate most on and try to create auspiciousness in the wealth and health corners of all its members.

The modern Tantric School is best known for its use in internal decorating. Represented by the Hong Kong master Lin Yun, it uses a method based on eight corners which adapts the trigrams of the *Book of Changes* (*Yijing*), an ancient classic of divination allegedly compiled by Confucius around 500 B.C.E. The *Book of Changes* is a fortune-telling manual that helps people determine the inherent tendencies in the course of nature and aids them in making good decisions by giving moral advice. It was adopted by the Chinese upper classes to provide personal readings for their official careers and family concerns, and has recently become popular in the West.

The system of the *Book of Changes* is based on yin and yang, symbolized by written lines: an unbroken line indicates yang, a broken line shows yin. The two lines, like the binary pattern at the base of computing, are combined two by two into four symbols: double yang, double yin, yang over yin, and yin over yang. In addition, the lines are also combined into eight symbols of three lines each, known as the eight trigrams (*bagua*) and linked symbolically with cosmic objects. They are: ☰ heaven (creative); ☷ earth (receptive), ☲ fire (clinging), ☵ water (deep), ☴ wind (gentle), ☱ lake (joyous), ☳ thunder (arousing), and ☶ mountain (still) (www.zhouyi.com).

Beyond this, the *Book of Changes* combines two trigrams each into figures consisting of six lines, the so-called sixty-four hexagrams. Each hexagram then comes with a divinatory text, an explanation of the image, a judgment, a commentary on the judgment, and a fortune for each individual line. A typical image explanation is, for example, "Clouds rise up to heaven, the image of waiting. Thus the superior man eats and drinks, is joyous and of good cheer" (Hex. 5), while a classic piece of advice in the judgment might be: "Waiting. If you are sincere, you have light and success. Perseverance brings good fortune; it furthers one to cross the great water" (Wilhelm, *I Ching*, 24–25; www.users.lmi.net/~tlc/iching).

The most common way to obtain a hexagram fortune from the *Book of Changes* is to throw three identical coins, in which head is designated yang and tail means yin. Yang counts 3, while yin counts 2. Throwing the three coins at any one time will result in the total number of either 6,

7, 8, or 9. These translate into lines: 9 = strong yang, 6 = strong yin, 7 = weak yang, and 8 = weak yin. After each throw, the line is written down and the hexagram is obtained from the bottom up. The strong lines, moreover, can change into their opposites (again from the bottom up), creating multiple hexagrams from one throw and allowing a longer-term prognosis.

> **Exercise:** Obtain a copy of the *Yijing* in translation (www.sacred-texts.com/ich) or go to www.facade.com/iching and divine a question, formulated in the format: "What if I did . . . ?" See whether the answer makes any sense.

Applying the eight trigrams of the *Book of Changes* to the house, eight corners are identified, signifying good fortune in specific areas of life. To find them, place the octagon with the bottom line on the front door. The system applies to any living space, always using the first access doorway as the baseline. In other words, your second floor may have a different orientation than your first floor; your bedroom and study each have their own set of corners.

Independent of where it is, each corner should be treated with care, kept free of clutter and dirt. To enhance its power, one can also place a suitable positive item in them, such as a bowl of coins, a fish bowl, or the picture of a waterfall in the money corner, a wedding picture or flowers in the marriage corner, and so on. The idea is that the corners are representative centers of *qi*-flow and their treatment enhances positive trends.

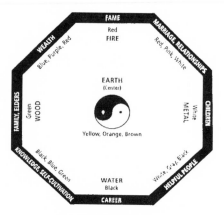

Fig. 23. The eight corners in the home.

Problems arise when the ground plan of the house is such that certain corners are missing or extraneous. Ideally the house should have an even ground plan. L-shaped houses are not recommended, since they miss one corner and have excess in another. Dormer windows and porches, on the other hand, additions to the basic ground plan, do not impact the *bagua*. If a corner is missing or in some other way impaired, various remedies can be used. The most common is the Fengshui mirror, a round mirror set in an octagonal frame that symbolizes the eight trigrams. It can be placed either on the inside or the outside of the house to reflect light and thus the flow of *qi* into an auspicious direction. Also, the planting of a tree or the placement of a lamp outside the house in the missing corner area can make up for the structural shortcoming.

For dark corners or hallways, crystals and wind-chimes are recommended. They reflect and disperse *qi* as light or sound, opening the area to good influences. Lights and plants are other remedies that can be placed to advantage. Various water ornaments, including fountains and aquariums, or pictures of rivers and waterfalls tend to symbolize the flow of money into the house and should be placed in the money corners. They are not as good in the relationship corner, where stability is preferred. To alleviate low ceilings or sharp edges in lofts, bamboo flutes and tassels can be hung. To make wide open spaces more comfortable and allow the *qi* to meander rather than rush, solid, strong objects, such as armchairs, rocks, or a statue might be placed.

In addition, all rooms should have the colors of the five phases present in one way or another, even if only in traces. Color schemes should use darker elements below and lighter elements above. White is not a preferred color in the Chinese world. Associated with the fall, it is the color of mourning and accordingly used sparingly. Modern Fengshui practitioners also see it as the color of intellect and analysis; they warn that too much white in a house will prevent people from making decisions. But off-white or various beige tones are highly suitable. Some colors are introduced through nature: green/blue is usually brought in through plants, while yellow/brown is represented in wooden floors or dark rugs. Red and black should be present, too, but not in overwhelming amounts, possibly in certain pieces of furniture or paintings.

Exercise: Pick a room or apartment and evaluate it in terms of Fengshui, examining its location in relation to the environment, the placement of furniture and objects in its corners, and the colors present.

Each room should be located and furnished to the best advantage. For example, the bedroom is best placed in the marriage or health corner. Not in direct line to the door, the bed should yet afford a clear view of the door (as should the desk in one's office). It should be neither too close to a window nor directly under a ceiling beam, neither in a wide-open area nor in a cramped, confined space. Also, the bedroom should be a refuge, a comforting and inviting space that enhances sensuality and encourages relaxation. Thus all things that remind the person of daily chores or the problems of the outside world should be removed. Mirrors, although usually beneficial in Fengshui, may be out of place in the bedroom since they enhance *qi* and potentially keep the room too active. Nor should there be any clutter or color combinations that might obstruct the *qi*. Everything in the room should either have a clear purpose or be there to enhance well-being and delight. Applying this to one's entire environment and all rooms in the house, the *qi* improves and so do the health, vigor, and good fortune of the family.

Further Readings

Collins, Terah Kathryn. 1996. *The Western Guide to Feng Shui*. Carlsbad, Calif.: Hay House.

Harper, Donald. 1978. "The Han Cosmic Board." *Early China* 4: 1-10.

Kingston, Karen. 1997. *Creating Sacred Space with Feng Shui*. New York: Broadway Books.

Kwok, Man-Ho, and Joanna O'Brien. 1995. *The Feng Shui Kit*. Tokyo: Tuttle.

Lip, Evelyn. 1995. *Feng Shui: Environments of Power. A Study of Chinese Architecture*. London: Academy Editions.

Oschman, James. 2000. *Energy Medicine: The Scientific Basis*. New York: Churchill Livingstone.

Rossbach, Sarah. 1983. *Feng Shui: The Chinese Art of Placement*. New York: Dutton.

Seaman, Gary. 1992. "Winds, Waters, Seeds, and Souls: Folk Concepts of Physiology and Etiology in Chinese Geomancy." In *Paths to Asian Medical Knowledge*, edited by Charles Leslie and Allan Young, 74-97. Berkeley: University of California Press.

Thompson, William Irvin, ed. 1987. *Gaia, a Way of Knowing: Political Implications of the New Biology*. Great Barrington, Mass: Lindisfarne Press.

Wilhelm, Richard. 1950. *The I Ching or Book of Changes*. Princeton: Princeton University Press.

Chapter 13
Food Cures and Diets

The *qi* of the outside world also enters the body and interacts with our inborn primordial *qi*. It does so first of all through food, giving value to the old adage that "you are what you eat." Thus, eating the right kind of food can cure the body while wrong or damaging food can make it ail. In East Asia, there are several ways in which food is used medically:

1. Food cures, also known as Chinese medicated diet or nutritional therapy, consist of ordinary food classified according to its healing properties and used for prevention and healing;

2. Macrobiotics, a Japanese adaptation of the Chinese food system, emphasizes whole foods, locally grown, and chewed thoroughly;

3. Daoist diet, for religious goals, involves the abstention from grain, increased herbal supplements, and periods of fasting.

Food cures use ordinary food stuffs and drinks for the prevention and cure of diseases. They employ everything people normally eat, but emphasize the food's medical and energetic qualities.

Documented since the third century B.C.E. and linked with the legendary founder of agriculture, the Divine Farmer (Shennong), they focus on prevention and cure, taking only a marginal interest in the alleviation of symptoms. This means that in some cases working on a problem with a change in diet may at first make symptoms more intense until a deeper, more permanent cure is effected. Still, Chinese nutritional therapy does not sub-

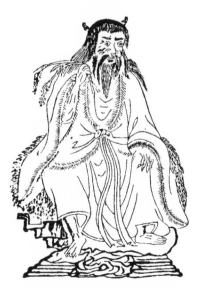

Fig. 24. Shennong, the Divine Farmer.

scribe to the dictum "good medicine tastes bitter" but tries to create tasty alternatives to habitual eating patterns.

The basic teaching of Chinese eating is to use clean and fresh foods, pure in color and clear in texture. Avoid anything old, moth-eaten, rotten, poor in quality, as well as anything processed, canned, or preserved. The more natural the food, the better. In this point, Chinese food cures are in perfect agreement with Western health food supporters. Then, however, the differences begin. Food in China is not classified on the basis of the food pyramid and its chemical constituents, such as carbohydrates, proteins, and fats, nor do they use calories or free radicals or other modern evaluation methods. Rather, the Chinese system arranges foods according to properties, flavors, and energetic movements. The most basic division is into yin and yang. Yin foods tend to grow in the earth and in dark, shady locations; they are sweet in flavor, fatty in consistence, and rich in potassium. Yang foods grow in air and sunshine; they are salty in flavor, lean in consistence, and rich in sodium. Yin foods include raw food, leafy vegetables, fish, and mellow tasting substances; they have a cooling, moisturizing, and decongesting effect, and promote fluid production while mitigating heat accumulation. Yang foods include anything fried, boiled, fatty, or spicy, as well as meats; they are warming, drying, and stimulating in nature, and as they absorb the cooking heat, they generate heat in the body and stimulate circulation.

Within this general system, food has three major properties:

1. stimulating (yang/heating/qi-enhancing)—apricots, barley, cherries, pineapple, plums, celery, coconut;

2. calming (yin/cooling/qi-reducing)—bananas, bean curd, cucumbers, eggplant, lettuce, mushrooms, pumpkins, tomatoes, watermelon;

3. neutral (neither yin nor yang/qi-maintaining)—apples, cabbage, carrots, papaya, grain, beans, eggs.

These properties are associated with the four seasons, with people's ages, and with particular mental states. Thus, foods eaten in spring should be stimulating and neutral; in summer, they should have a calming and cooling effect; in the fall, they should serve to retain fluid (more meats); and in winter they should stimulate and warm the body. In other words, food is used to balance the energetic pattern of the seasons, and people should eat yin foods in yang times and yang foods in yin times. However, at all times one should avoid raw and ice-cold substances, since their yin properties deplete the system, weaken the spleen, and harm the small intestine.

Another modification of the food intake is according to age. Young people tend to be warmer, more energetic, and more yang in quality, while older folks have increased yin. Small children, being the most yang, often crave sweets to mellow their yang-*qi*. Older people, on the contrary, tend to like meats, stews, and warming foods to counteract their yin-nature. Beyond this, food also has an effect on the mental attitude. If we lack in confidence and depend much on others, more yang food may be indicated; if we tend to be aggressive, assertive, and stubborn, a mellowing yin-rich diet would be beneficial. Overall, yang foods increase valor and energy, while yin foods will have a calming and slowing effect (see Craze and Jay, *Cooking for Long Life*, 19, 23).

A more subtle Chinese classification of food, which follows upon the yin-yang division, is according to the five flavors:

1. spicy or pungent (metal) — linked with lungs and large intestine; induces perspiration and promotes *qi* and blood circulation: green onions, chives, cloves, parsley, peppermint, cinnamon, chili, curry;

2. sweet (earth) — associated with spleen and stomach; slows down acute symptoms and neutralizes toxicity: string beans, cherries, chestnuts, bananas, honey, watermelon;

3. sour (wood) — linked with liver and gall bladder problems; obstructs movement; useful in controlling diarrhea and excessive fluids, such as perspiration: apples, grapefruit, lemons, pears, plums, mangoes, vinegar;

4. bitter (fire) — related to the heart and small intestine; reduces body heat, dries body fluids, and expels excess liquids, may induce diarrhea: hops, lettuce, radish leaves;

5. salty (water) — associated with kidney and bladder issues; warms the body, softens hardness; treats tuberculosis of lymph nodes and other symptoms involving hardening of muscles or glands: pickled vegetables. (See www.foodsn herbs.com)

The five tastes should be evenly balanced in every meal to stimulate the organs properly and eliminate wayward *qi*. The *qi*-flow in the meridians can be regulated by using food much like acupuncture points, examining a given imbalance in terms of excess and deficiency, analyzing it in relation to the cycles of the five phases, then tonifying the son or draining the mother, depending on the situation.

Next, all foods also have specific energetic effects, described in terms of temperature:

cold	cool	neutral	warm	hot
effects on		effects on	effects on	
stomach yin		center	spleen yang	
lung yin		triple heater	kidney yang	
liver yin			heart yang	
kidney yin			liver yang	

Fig. 25 . The temperature qualities of food.

While most foods naturally have a temperature quality, some also change depending on their state. Thus, for example, raw wheat has a tendency to be cool and neutral, supporting the center of the body; when sprouted it becomes cold and acquires a slightly pungent taste, serving to alleviate heated conditions; as cooked porridge, wheat is mainly neutral and sweet, enhancing *qi*; and when baked as wheat flour, it obtains a warm temperature and aids in treating cool or cold body conditions (Engelhardt and Hempen, *Chinesische Diätetik*, 411).

The different temperature qualities of food are intrinsically related to the five phases and their corresponding organs and meridians. For example, a liver weakened by too much yin food can develop an imbalance with the spleen and may cause it to overwork. This in turn may lead to an overflow of acidic secretions in the stomach, felt as heartburn and acid reflux. On the other hand, the warming and cooling qualities of food can be used to modify already existing imbalances, increasing the *qi* through warm or hot food in a weakened meridian or depleting it through cool or cold things in one that shows signs of excess or inflammation.

Another way to examine the quality of food in the Chinese system is by looking at its dominant movement:

1. outwards: induces perspiration and reduces fever; use in summer; spicy or sweet (pepper, ginger);

2. inwards: eases bowel movements and abdominal swelling; use in winter; bitter or salty (lettuce, clams, crabs, seaweed);

3. upwards: relieves diarrhea, prolapsed anus or uterus, falling stomach; use in spring; spicy, sweet, or bitter (apricots, celery, cherries, grapes, olives, potatoes, peanuts, rice);

4. downwards: relieves vomiting, hiccupping, and asthma; use in fall; sweet or sour (apples, bananas, cucumbers, grapefruit, lettuce, peaches, strawberries).

Beyond these, there are also glossy foods that facilitate digestion (honey, spinach) and obstructive foods which slow it down (guava, olives). For example: to disperse cold, use ginger or wine; to improve the appetite, eat green or red pepper or ham; to induce a bowel movement, take castor beans or sesame oil; to reduce fever, eat star fruit or water chestnuts; and to relieve pain, take honey or squash. Also for a headache due to increased heat, use cooling and downward moving foods, such as wheat, beans, bamboo sprouts, radish, spinach, and tomatoes. To help in cases of blood and *qi* stagnation (angina pectoris), use foods that stimulate and move blood and *qi*, including leeks, onions, vinegar, crabs, and small quantities of wine. For erectile dysfunction, often caused by a depletion of kidney-*qi*, take walnuts, cinnamon, anchovies, mussels, mutton, and game (Engelhardt and Hempen, *Chinesische Diätetik*, 576-85). In all cases, the ideal is to create a diet that balances the body's tendencies and symptoms in movement as well as flavors and energetic tendencies.

> **Exercise:** Create a sample menu for someone with a cold-induced fever that affects the lung meridian. Then try one for someone who suffers from insomnia and nervousness due to liver heat rising.

Because of its strong emphasis on balance which includes also the need for hot, energy-giving yang foods, Chinese medicine does not support a vegetarian diet. Vegetarians eat too many cooling, yin foods, thus depleting their *qi* to levels suitable only for recluses who are not physically active. By the same token, the addition of fish to a vegetarian diet, although it provides protein according to the Western system, will not increase yang, since fish is a cool food that relates to water and therefore yin. On the other hand, a diet overly heavy in proteins and meat is not beneficial either, since highly caloric, strong yang foods, may deplete the body's *qi* by causing certain organs to overwork and creating deficiencies in others. It is best, therefore, to eat some meat, but not too much and if possible organic, healthy specimens free of hormones and stimulants.

Not only the choice of food is important, however, but also how it is prepared and eaten. Food should be viewed as a precious gift from nature, a treasure trove of health and vitality, and accordingly treated with gratitude and respect. Cooking should be done in a quiet and peaceful atmosphere, with plenty of time and enjoyment. The cook's mind should be relaxed and full of giving, loving vibrations, since his or her attitude will influence how the food works and tastes. As Craze and Jay say, "As you cook, breathe deeply and slowly. Work gently as if holding a new-born baby. Keep harsh noises to a minimum" (*Cooking for Long Life*, 36). Similarly, food should not be eaten on the run or while engaged in other activities. Sit down calmly; take time to enjoy the looks, smells, and tastes of the food; eat slowly and develop a sense of peace and wholeness through the act of eating. All this contributes to a greater sense of harmony and will aid the digestion and *qi*-flow of the body.

Beyond cooking and eating consciously, Chinese food cures also recommend the frequent consumption of tea, especially green tea. Mentioned already in texts that go back to around 800 B.C.E., tea has always been a mainstay of Chinese culture. Botanically a member of the *Camellia* family, tea grows as various shrubs that can reach fifty feet in height and commonly bear shiny leaves whose ends form pointed, spear-like tips. Picked and dried or roasted, and occasionally mixed with blossoms or flowers, the leaves are prepared to make different teas. The white or pale green variety uses them almost raw, while black or red tea applies them more roasted or fermented. Tea can contain large amounts of caffeine in all forms, and commonly has been used in religious institutions to keep monks and nuns from falling asleep during meditation periods.

In classical Chinese literature, tea is almost exclusively described as bitter, but it has also been linked with the sweet flavor. Its medical benefits include the ability to increase blood flow, heighten awareness, speed elimination, prevent tooth decay, aid digestion, cleanse the skin, alleviate joint pain, and generally prolong life (Blofeld, *Chinese Art of Tea*, 144). It is also a way to ingest all five phases in one fell swoop: earth through the bowl's ceramics, metal in the kettle, water as its base, wood in the plant from which it grew, and fire in the heating. Western studies, too, have shown that especially green tea with low caffeine contains antioxidants which bind harmful free radicals. Drinking it regularly can prevent cell mutation in tumors, promote healthy arteries, reduce cholesterol, release toxins, aid digestion, increase metabolism, and control bacteria.

Both food and tea are accorded great importance in Chinese society. Wherever one goes, tea is served, and people carry portable mugs; whenever people come together, there is food. The Chinese tend to spend much money on high-quality food and take hours to prepare dishes and enjoy their meals. Often factories and schools close for three hours over lunch, so that everybody can go home to prepare and eat a proper meal. Food is not bought in advance, but people go to their local market to purchase the freshest local foods, best adapted to the local weather and meant to help their consumer to thrive locally as well. As Kate Townsend reports:

> During our last trip to China, we were fed wonderful meals three times a day. Typical meals included twelve or sixteen different dishes at lunch and dinner. The manner in which we ate—as a group, taking moderate amounts of a variety of food over the course of an hour—satisfied not only the five phases of taste, but also the spiritual nourishment of sharing meals with good company and good conversation.

> Despite eating way more frequently than I do at home, in two weeks I probably lost twelve pounds. It was a great opportunity to recognize what food and nourishment really mean. Our food was prepared with the freshest ingredients and had minimal (if any) amounts of sugar, wheat, and dairy. (personal communication)

With their more balanced approach to food the Chinese eat a much healthier diet than modern Americans. As Linda Prout emphasizes, statistics have shown that the Chinese "eat about 30 percent more calories than we do and skip the gym workout, yet they are 25 percent thinner than we are. On top of that, the Chinese have 17 times fewer cases of heart disease, one-fifth the rate of breast cancer, and less than half the instances of colon cancer we do. Their cholesterol levels are about half ours" (*Live in the Balance*, 9).

Exercise: Describe the typical diet and eating habits in your life and society. How does it account for your and your family's health or disease? How could and should it be altered to create more harmony?

Given this situation, it is not surprising that Chinese food cures in various forms have been introduced not only as slimming diets but also as a form of healing in the West. Most popular among them is a method developed in Japan and known as macrobiotics, which literally means "big life," referring to its broad perspective. Its founder, George Ohsawa (1893-1966), in 1909 contracted tuberculosis and was told that he would die soon. Trying to avoid this, he studied a book by Sagen Ishizuka called *The Curative Method of Diet* and began to eat accordingly. He consumed only natural foods and beverages and made whole grains the backbone of his diet. After he cured himself, he taught the method to others. His main disciples were Herman Aikawa and Michio Kushi. In 1949, the latter brought the practice to the U.S. where he gave lectures, conducted workshops, wrote books, and founded centers in Boston and San Francisco. He educated wide segments of the population on the relationship between diet, lifestyle, and disease, and with his whole-food nutrition method was successful in curing numerous degenerative diseases, including terminal cases (see www.macrobiotics.org).

Macrobiotics is based on the cosmology of yin and yang in relationship to the Dao, which here is described as Infinity. Infinity manifests itself in the complementary forces yin and yang, which are endless in change and transformation. Yin represents centrifugality; yang represents centripetality. Together they produce energy and all phenomena. They both attract and repel each other and constantly change into one another. Nothing ever is solely yin or solely yang, and one has to maintain the proper balance between them for continued health and prosperity.

To find this balance, one should eat organically grown, whole, and local foods that are in season. One should listen to the body, undertake regular exercise, and keep stress levels low. To eat specifically in the macrobiotic way, one should create meals that contain one part yang to five parts yin. This ratio is found naturally in whole grains, especially in brown rice, which should make up half of one's diet. The next quarter should be vegetables, chosen according to the one-to-five ratio of yin and yang. Vegetables should not be boiled but steamed or lightly sautéed and eaten cooked for the most part (20%); only a small portion should be consumed raw or as pickles (5%). The remaining quarter of the daily food is divided equally among beans, seaweed, condiments/pickles, soups, and beverages (Kushi and Esko, *Holistic Health*).

Macrobiotic practitioners avoid caffeine, alcohol, chocolate, sugar, meat, dairy, mints, and sodas; anything canned, frozen, or irradiated; as well as all artificially colored, preserved, sprayed, or chemically treated foods. They drink comparatively little water on the assumption that a vegetable-based, low-sodium diet allows the body to absorb sufficient liquid from food, whereas too much water will create an excess of yin and lead to unhealthy conditions. Also, once healthy foods are chosen, the preparation should not destroy them. For this reason, macrobiotic cooks prefer natural oils, rice paste, or beans as oils and use only natural utensils such as unglazed pottery or earthenware, wooden spatulas and strainers. Meals are an important time, during which the focus is entirely on the food. Chewing should be patient and conscious, and a portion of the stomach should always remain empty.

If undertaken as healing therapy, macrobiotics detoxifies the body, supports its self-healing ability, and enhances the immune system. It increases the functioning of the organs and creates natural stabilization. It has been shown to improve or cure arthritis, heart disease, hypertension, hepatitis, migraines, diabetes, digestive problems, autoimmune disorders, allergies, obesity, and even cancer. It is not merely a diet, however, but involves a complete change in lifestyle, spending more time preparing and eating food and becoming more conscious of one's relationship to nature and Infinity. It may sound expensive but is in fact quite affordable, since the amount of food one consumes is considerably less than in a diet that relies on processed foods. The body, after all, eats *until* it gets the nourishment it needs: the more one consumes calories without nutrients, the longer and the more one has to eat.

The third form of Chinese diet is the Daoist way of eating. Traditionally Daoists have divided diet into three levels: eating food, herbs, and *qi*. That is to say, while still in ordinary society, Daoist laymen and priests follow the rules of Chinese food cures and eat everything while paying close attention to energetic potencies and seasonal influences (Saso, *Taoist Cookbook*). Then, as they develop in spiritual potency or join a monastic community, they gradually move beyond ordinary food, eat a vegetarian diet, and take more herbs and plant substances. Eventually, as immortality practices set in, even the herbs are no longer needed and the body is maintained through the intake of *qi* alone—through breathing exercises, swallowing the saliva, and meditations.

While most Daoists today are still eating, the goal for ancient practitioners was to move away from food toward *qi*. To do so, they undertook a practice known as *bigu* or "abstention from grain." *Bigu* begins with an avoidance of meat and alcohol, matching similar Buddhist rules but with a different motivation. Buddhists avoid meat because killing a living being, even if done by someone else, creates bad karma; similarly drinking alcohol leads to intoxication and may cause behavior that is harmful to others and brings about karmic burdens. Ancient Daoists avoided meat and alcohol not because of karma but because of their high yang-quality which would create obstructions to spiritual transformation.

In addition, Daoists in ancient China also avoided the five grains—rice, millet, barley, wheat, and beans—the staple of ordinary people. There are several reasons for this. On a physiological level, Daoists believed that cooking things is a form of processing and thus decay. The word *lan* in Chinese means both "cooked" and "putrefied," "rotten." According to Daoist understanding, meat decomposes in the intestines, grain rots in the stomach, and digestion is nothing but a form of decay that causes death. Rather than live on food that decays, they preferred to use herbs and plants that stayed whole and eventually did away with eating altogether and depended on the intake of pure, cosmic *qi*. A more mythological expression of the same idea was that grains in the body supported the continued presence of the Three Deathbringers, the demonic parasites who feed on decay and are eager for the body to die so they can devour it. To attain long life, Daoists contended, the Deathbringers had to be starved, and a good way to do so was to avoid grain.

Ancient Daoists accordingly ate fruits, nuts, mushrooms, and vegetables, then replaced these with elixirs of herbs, minerals, and metals, and eventually lived on pure *qi* through breathing exercises and meditations. Their basic tendency of avoiding cooked food matches the modern trend toward raw food, a movement which proposes a diet consisting of three quarters raw and one quarter cooked foods. Proponents of this argue that cooking or preserving food eliminates large amounts of vitamins and minerals and that any food heated over 116 degrees loses all enzymes and protein structure, so that the food actually takes good agents out of the body. Pasteurizing milk destroys three quarters of the milk protein; altered, partially hydrogenated fats can become lethal compounds, unlike whole fats, as found in nuts, virgin olive oil, and flaxseed oil (Kenton and Kenton, *Raw Energy*).

Exercise: Go to www.livingnutrition.com; www.sunorganic.com; www.fresh-network.com; www.TheRawWorld.com; or www.rawfamily.com and find recipes for a day of raw food. Reflect on how different this is from the macrobiotic diet. If the two were your only choices, which one would you pick and why?

The positive effects of a raw food diet are numerous. Adherents claim that it boosts lymphocyte production, empowers the immune system, and contains enzymes that aid digestion. It also delays the aging process, increases oxygen consumption, and leads to more vitality, energy, and athletic ability. Beyond that, it heightens the senses, increases sensitivity to alcohol, tobacco, and drugs, and improves sexuality and aesthetic sensibility. It aids weight loss, eases allergies (often caused by food toxins), helps cure addictions, can reduce tumor size, and help cancer recovery. It provides all eight of the twenty-two essential amino acids that must come from outside sources (especially through green leafy vegetables, pumpkin seeds, almonds, and fruits), increases flexibility and brain function through essential vegetable fats, and prevents diseases caused by pathogenic bacteria in meats and dairy.

The different schools in the Chinese understanding of diets and health agree that diet is an essential factor in creating and maintaining good health and that foods can be divided into yin and yang categories and classified according to their energetic properties. They all agree that it is best to use natural, whole foods and that with a healthy diet it is not necessary to drink lots of water. However, they disagree about the use of meat, alcohol, and grain as well as about the degree of cooking. Traditional Chinese food cures make use of everything and insist on cooking things. Macrobiotics avoid meat and alcohol but insist on lots of grain and extensive cooking. Raw food and *bigu* followers avoid all grain, meat, and alcohol and prefer foods uncooked. The variety of methods allows followers of the dietary path to tailor a specific mixture of foods and cooking techniques suitable to their personal tastes and health situation.

Further Readings:

Blofeld, John. 1985. *The Chinese Art of Tea*. Boston: Shambhala.

Butt, Gary and Frena Bloomfield. 1985. *Harmony Rules: The Chinese Way of Health Through Food*. York Beach, Minn.: Samuel Weiser.

Counihan, Carole M. 1999. *The Anthropology of Food and Body*. New York: Routledge.

Craze, Richard, and Roni Jay. 2001. *Cooking for Long Life: The Tao of Food*. New York: Sterling Publishing.

Engelhardt, Ute, and Carl-Hermann Hempen. 1997. *Chinesische Diätetik*. Munich: Urban & Schwarzenberg.

Kakuzo, Okakura. 1956: *The Book of Tea*. Boston: Tuttle.

Kenton, Leslie, and Susannah Kenton. 1984. *Raw Energy*. New York: Warner Books.

Kushi, Michio, and Edward Esko. 1993. *Holistic Health through Macrobiotics*. New York: Japan Publications.

Lu, Henry C. 1986. *Chinese System of Food Cures: Prevention and Remedies*. New York: Sterling Publishing.

Ni, Maoshing, and Cathy McNease. 1987. *The Tao of Nutrition*. Los Angeles: Seven Star Communication Group.

Nison, Paul. 2001. *The Raw Life: Becoming Natural in an Unnatural World*. New York: 343 Publishing.

Pitchford, Paul. 1993. *Healing with Whole Foods: Oriental Traditions and Modern Nutrition*. Berkeley: North Atlantic Books.

Prout, Linda. 2000. *Live in the Balance*. New York: Marlowe.

Romano, Rita. 1997. *Dining in the Raw*. New York: Kensington Publishers.

Saso, Michael. 1994. *A Taoist Cookbook*. Boston: Charles E. Tuttle.

Chapter 14

The Chinese Pharmacopoeia

In addition to food as a form of absorbing and regulating *qi*, herbs play an important part in Chinese health and long life practice. They can be self-administered and taken as dietary supplements or prescribed by a professional, either as a purely herbal treatment or in addition to acupuncture. The most effective use of herbs is in a clinical setting, where not only single herbs are prescribed but also compounds made up of five, ten, or more ingredients. Chinese pharmacological manuals list over 2,000 substances, about 530 of which are still commonly used. Not all come from plants; mineral and animal products are also well represented.

Herbal medicines vary according to local ingredients, symptom interpretation, and the matching of herbs to illnesses. However, all practitioners agree on the concept of root versus branch treatment. That is to say, they can either address the root, the underlying cause of the imbalance, or treat the branch, the obvious symptoms. Since herbal medicines are ingested and work systemically, the effect is synchronous and they can target only symptom at a time. In this regard they differ from acupuncture, physical manipulation, and Qigong therapy, where one treatment can have stages that address different concerns. On the other hand, practitioners adjust the formula as the patient's symptoms change, never allowing a long-term use of the same compound.

Chinese medicinal drug culture is traditionally known as pharmacopoeia or *materia medica* (*bencao*; saturn.ihp.sinica.tw/~bencao/index.htm). Historically, the first source on herbal remedies is the *Recipes for Fifty-two Ailments* (*Wushier bingfang*), found among the Mawangdui manuscripts of 168 B.C.E. The text includes 283 concoctions for fifty-two ailments. In outlook, it presents a harmonious blend of magic and the medical arts, with the idea that sickness is caused by microcosmic imbalances in the body and harmony can be restored through medicines and therapeutic techniques as well as through exorcisms against demons.

The second major work on Chinese herbs is the treatise *On Cold-Induced Disorders* (*Shanghan lun*; trl. Mitchell, Ye, and Wiseman 1999) of the third century C.E. The work was inspired by a large epidemic that devastated the country. Its original author Zhang Zhongjing interpreted the epidemic as being caused by the invasion of cold into the body. Symptoms vary as the body fights this. First there are cold symptoms, such as shivers, runny nose, tight neck muscles, cold hands and feet, and so on. Then, as the cold pathogen worms its way deeper, the visible signs shift to hot presentation, such as fevers, dry mouth, vomiting, sweat, and the like. Since the invader is cold in nature, the body responds with heating up. Following Zhang's premise, the physician Wang Shuhe expanded the treatise and developed Zhang's basic system by adding the eight diagnostic patterns and linking herbal compounds with symptoms, creating a first systematic application of Chinese herbs.

Their first overall classification is found in *The Divine Farmer's Materia Medica* (*Shennong bencao jing*), compiled by the Daoist Tao Hongjing (456-536). The work contains 365 drug recipes and classifies them according to three levels: lower-level or crude drugs that consist of only one ingredient; medium-level or drug formulas, which include several crude drugs combined; and top-level or more potent drugs, described as elixirs and designed to transform the body toward immortality. This classification stands in contrast to modern categories which focus on organ functions and the invasion of pathogenic factors. Later works deal not only with herbs, which they divide into various new categories, but also show a deep appreciation of longevity practices. The most prominent among them is the *Organized Materia Medica* (*Bencao gangmu*; trl. Stuart 1976) by the physician Li Shizhen (1518-1593).

Chinese herbs are grown today on specialized farms. Collected and dried, they are delivered to traditional pharmacies, where patients receive a mixture of ingredients to take home and boil. This decoction from original materials is the most potent form of Chinese herbs. Slightly less powerful are powders and pills, for which the herbs are broken up through pounding, grating, mincing, or flaking and further processed by boiling, burning, or steaming. The resulting substances are then powdered or formed into pills, which patients take with water. Alternatively, the substances are liquified by being mixed with alcohol, vinegar, and the like to create a tincture or syrup which is often quite tasty. As a final alternative, the herbal compound is fried in lard or mixed with oil to form a liniment or ointment. Applied externally, they are often also put on sticky plasters, helpful for muscle tension and injuries.

As regards their functioning, herbs in China are classified in similar ways as foods, i.e., according to properties, flavors, and actions. This contrasts sharply with Western classifications which tend to examine chemical constituents and their relation to body chemistry. Being materialistic and reductionistic in outlook, Western approaches to herbs look for actual physical substances within the plants and tend to confine their explanations for the herbs' effects to those few substances. Their main concern is the mechanism of how and why these substances work the way they do. A more recent way of classification combines the Western and Eastern approaches and divides herbs into five categories, according to their dominant function: elimination, restoration, drainage, regulation, and symptom treatment (Holmes, *Energetics*).

In China, the major properties of herbs are cooling or warming, i.e., clearing heat, removing toxicity, and nourishing yin versus dispersing cold, warming the organs, and supporting yang. They come in the same five flavors as foods, i.e., spicy (ginger, mint, pepper), sweet (licorice, dates, ginseng), bitter (rhubarb, watercress), sour (lemon, crabapple, orange peel), and salty (seaweed). Their effects are stimulating, warming/relaxing, detoxifying, refreshing, and softening, and they treat syndromes connected to the matching organs. Typically the properties and flavors of herbs go together, i.e., hot drugs tend to be spicy or salty. However, it also happens that two drugs of the same flavor have different properties. For example, both ephedra (*mahuang*) and mint are classified as spicy, but ephedra warms while mint cools.

> **Exercise:** Look up two or three common Western herbs like chamomile, echinacea, or St. John's wort, and classify them in terms of properties and taste. How do they fit into the Chinese system? Does their use match this understanding?

The third classification of Chinese herbs is according to their actions:

1. Lifting—going or sending upward, invigorate *qi* and raise yang, used for diseases in the upper body and exterior, and those with a downward tendency (diarrhea, prolapsed uterus).

2. Floating—going outward or sending to the surface, elevates yang, relieves exterior symptoms by dispelling superficial wind and cold, facilitates resuscitation.

3. Lowering—going down or sending down, lowers yang, used for diseases in the lower part of the body or interior (constipation) and for those moving upward (headache).

4. Sinking—going inside or purging, used in conjunction with lowering drugs, controls excess of yang, clears heat, removes dampness, lowers adverse *qi*-flow, relieves cough and asthma, tranquilizes mind, improves digestion.

Within this overall framework, certain Chinese herbs are taken singly and used as dietary supplements. They include honey (sweet, warming), licorice (tonifying and detoxifying), ginseng (major *qi* tonic), cinnamon (warming), garlic (increases heat), ginger (warms interior), gingko (respiration, memory), and citrus peel (indigestion, hiccups) (www.acupuncture.com/herbology/herbind.htm).

The best known and most classical Chinese herb is ginseng. It is already described in the *The Divine Farmer's Materia Medica*:

> Ginseng is a tonic for the five organs. It helps quiet the material soul, stabilize the spirit soul, prevent fear, expel wayward *qi*, brighten the eyes to improve vision, and open the heart to benefit comprehension. If taken for longer periods, it will invigorate the entire body and prolong life.

Ginseng is a deciduous plant that grows to a height of ten feet and bears leaves on each stem. Its root looks like a human body with various extremities and has from early times been associated with human vitality. Chemically it contains saponins known as ginsenosides, supporters of the immune system, and comes in over thirty types. Today its best-known varieties are Korean/Siberian and American ginseng.

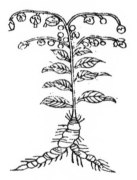

Fig. 26. The ginseng root.

Siberian ginseng increases *qi*. It helps with stress and weakness, has strong antioxidant properties, and stimulates the production of nitrous oxide as well as other immune-system components. It can prevent respiratory infections, reduce inflammation, lower blood sugar, and increase blood flow to the brain. In this latter function, it helps with concentration (ADD/ADHD) and eases depression. It can also stimulate the production of testosterone and help with erectile dysfunction. It is a popular drug for athletes who use it to increase performance, bolster the immune system, ease fatigue, and reduce stress. Ginseng has also been shown effective for diabetes, since it lowers the glycemic response after carbohydrate consumption. Its most exciting use is in the fight against cancer. It stimulates B cells, which are depleted in chronic leukemia, multiple myeloma, and ovarian carcinoma (Rister, *Japanese Herbal Medicine*, 106). However, its long-term use can lead to heart palpitations and agitation. As with all herbs, it is best to consult with a trained practitioner before introducing it into a heath regimen.

American ginseng is a smaller version of the Asian variety. Already used among Native Americans, it has a bitter-sweet flavor and cooling properties. Its main effect is to strengthen the body's yin or constraining functions and to lower fevers. It helps in respiratory ailments, recovery from disease, and liver overload. Especially people whose livers have suffered from years of abuse through the consumption of fatty, spicy foods and alcohol find relief through American ginseng. It, too, should be taken with care and not over long periods (Fulder, *Book of Ginseng*).

Another Chinese classic is gingko, also found in the early literature. It was first introduced to Europe in the 1700s and has since become widely popular. Both the fan-shaped leaves and little round nuts are used, but for different purposes. Seen in China as a dry agent that fights dampness, the leaves release an extract that contains flavenoids and terpenoids which inhibit a chemical called PAF (platelet activating factor). As a result, gingko leaf extract keeps the muscles from contracting and helps in cases of heart attack, stroke, and poor circulation in the legs. Its best publicized use is in cases of memory loss, ADD, dementia, and Alzheimer's disease. It speeds the assimilation of glucose in the brain and increases blood flow to it, while enhancing a memory-supporting chemical called acetylcholine (Rister, *Japanese Herbal Medicine*, 101).

Gingko nuts, on the other hand, relieve respiratory and reproductive problems. Bitter-sweet in taste, they strengthen the lungs, loosen phlegm, relieve asthma, tuberculosis, and also help in cases of frequent urination and vaginal discharge. In China, gingko has also been seen as a longevity drug that will reverse the aging process and will improve vision and hearing, a feature that Westerners link with its antioxidant properties. On the downside, gingko can cause mild stomach pains, an occasional headache, and allergic reactions. It should not be used with blood thinners, such as aspirin, since there is a danger of hemorrhaging (Halpern, *Gingko*).

The most common Chinese medicinal herb, used in cooking and for healing is garlic. Originally from Central Asia, it was well known already in the ancient world and today is grown everywhere. Available in fresh bulbs, as oil-based extracts, dried powders, and pills, it kills internal parasites and is known as the poor man's antibiotic. It contains many natural antioxidants, anti-clotting agents, and detoxifiers, released as the phytochemical allicin when a clove is crushed or cooked. Also containing various sulfur compounds which inhibit platelets in the blood from adhering to one another, garlic has been shown to lower cholesterol, protect the heart, and serve as an anti-inflammatory and pain-relieving remedy. It is good for colds, asthma, diabetes, yeast infections, and many other ailments. It has also, for many years, been known to reduce the risk of cancer, especially of the breast, colon, larynx, and stomach. On the negative side, garlic can lead to blood thinning and should be avoided before or after surgery. Very high doses will also irritate the intestines, not to mention other people.

Like garlic, ginger comes originally from Asia and is now grown everywhere. Already Confucius was known for not removing the ginger from his food, thus absorbing its healing properties; and Shakespeare says in *Love's Labours Lost*: ". . . had I but one penny in the world thou shouldst have it to buy ginger-bread." About one-third of the 113 herbal recipes in *On Cold-Induced Disorders* and about two-thirds of all modern compounds include ginger. It is the root of a tropical plant that grows two feet high and is available raw as well as in powdered and capsule forms. Its active ingredients are terpenoids, gingerols, and shogoals. Its main action is the relief of dampness and chill, and it is said to "rescue devastated yang" (Rister, *Japanese Herbal Medicine*, 56). Boiled in water and made into a tea, it helps colds. Small doses of ginger also settle the stomach; prevent motion sickness, nausea, and side-effects of other drugs; alleviate morning sickness (with a delay of 48 hours); warm the body; stop bleeding; make the heart beat more strongly; and reduce fevers and pains. For the most part, ginger is beneficial. However, if taken over long periods of time, it can increase bile and acid secretion and may irritate the stomach.

Radish (daikon) is the yin counterpart to ginger. Originally Chinese but now grown everywhere, it is cooling and fresh, tastes sweet and pungent, and is generally nourishing for the body. Like ginger, it strengthens the spleen and the stomach, opens their channels, and enhances digestion. In addition, it is beneficial for the lungs and helps in infections and tuberculosis. It lowers the rush of *qi*, decreases phlegm, and detoxifies the body. It tastes good and can be easily added to soups, stir-fries, and salads. Its juice, pressed from the fresh plant, is good against thirst, nosebleeds, and oral lesions (Fang, "Anwendung von Rettich").

Less well known but taken to good effect and second only to ginger in its commonality, especially in herbal compounds, is licorice root. Growing everywhere, the plant is a woody-stemmed perennial that grows to a height of six feet and has creamy white flowers. When three or four years old, its roots are dug up, dried, and fried either plain or with honey. Licorice is considered the "emergency herb" of the Chinese pharmacopoeia, since it is most effective in treating acute symptoms or infections.

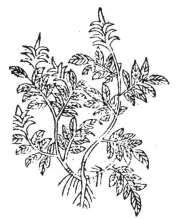

Fig. 27. The licorice plant.

The intravenous injection of the licorice compound glycyrrhizin into AIDS patients has resulted in remarkable improvements, and it is commonly used in the treatment of hepatitis. More generally, licorice root tonifies the digestive tract and is helpful in both hot and cold conditions. This universal power plus its intense sweetness (about fifty times that of table sugar) makes it an ideal harmonizer of other herbs, and licorice is accordingly found in numerous Asian compounds (Rister, *Japanese Herbal Medicine*, 66).

Exercise: Go to the web (www.tmcbasics.com/materiamedical.htm; www.rmhiherbal.org) or find a book on Chinese herbs and look up the nature and use of three herbs of your choice, like cinnamon, dates, Chinese angelica (danggui/tang-kuei), ephedra, or hawthorn. What are the properties of these substances? What are their healing effects? How commonly are they used?

Beyond single herbs that can be applied both medically and as dietary supplements, Chinese health practice relies heavily on formulas or compounds. Used for healing rather than as a supplement, they are prescribed by professionals and come either as raw herbs for decoction or prepackaged as powders and pills. Formulas often follow the pattern of the four responsible roles, designating the lead and secondary herbs. According to this, one herb or group of herbs is the "emperor," i.e., the primary active ingredient which is most potent and whose action is geared most strongly toward alleviating the ailment. Another herb or group functions as the "minister," i.e., as secondary power that assists and reinforces the action of the "emperor," providing complementary benefits. A third aspect of the compound is the "assistant," a slightly less central function that counteracts potential negative side-effects of the other herbs and neutralizes those potencies in "emperor" and "minister" not needed for the ailment. Fourth and finally, there is the "servant," a general factotum whose task it is to harmonize the actions of the other herbs and promote their rapid absorption into qi, blood, and organs— often licorice, as noted above (www.rxlist.com/chinese.htm).

To give a few examples, to relieve tension headaches, people take Evodia Concoction (Wujuyu tang), which contains evodia, ginseng, Chinese dates, and fresh ginger to the effect of enhancing qi and releasing fatigue. The common cold is best treated with Cold Effective Pills (Ganmao ling wan), based on esatis, evodia, chrysanthemum flowers, vitex fruit, lanicer flower, and menthol crystals. It helps the immune system neutralize and eliminate the invading wind pathogens, relieves acute flare-ups, and reduces fever. Another prominent cold remedy is Honeysuckle Tablets (Yinjiao pian), containing honeysuckle flower and forsythia fruit with burdock, mint, soya seeds, and licorice (Elias and Ketcham, *Five Elements of Self-Healing*, 191-92).

In cases of asthma, a convenient and highly potent remedy is found in Asthma Relief Pills (Pingchuan wan). They support lungs and kidneys, break up phlegm, and stop coughs. They contain armeniaca as emperor, attended by codonopsis root, licorice, eleagnus fruit, ficus leaf, citrus peel, and cordyceps fungus among others. For digestive problems, take Harmony Preserve Pills (Baohe wan), which contain hawthorn, pinella root, tangerine peel, forsythia fruit, wheat sprouts, and radish seeds. They strengthen the spleen qi and enhance yang in the body.

These are just a few examples of readily available medicines in the modern Chinese pharmacopoeia. Many more herbs are being used by practitioners who will often also prescribe custom-made combinations to match the specific symptoms and energetic patterns of their patients. These combinations as much as the pill formulas do not rely solely on vegetable materials, but often also contain minerals and animal ingredients. Among the latter, the most common are parts of cockroaches, geckos, spiders, locusts, centipedes, earth worms, and other crawly creatures as well as snakes, frogs, and fish, each valued for its specific potency. For example, a popular patent formula called Gecko Tonifying Pills (Gejie dabu wan) has desiccated gecko lizard as its emperor, supported by seven plant substances. It is excellent for strengthening *qi* and blood, enhancing vitality and the immune system.

Beyond these rather common animals, parts of certain protected species are highly sought after among Chinese pharmacists and patients. This, of course, is illegal since their harvest is leading to the extinction of the animal. However, the laws tend not to be very well enforced and there is a large and highly profitable black market. Examples include:

> deer antlers: salty, increase yang, libido (aphrodisiac);
>
> rhinoceros horns: salty, eliminate excess heat and toxins (heart, liver, stomach);
>
> seal kidneys: salty, strengthen yang, warm kidneys, relieve impotence (kidneys);
>
> turtle shells: sweet, eliminate excess heat and toxicity, cool blood, stabilize nerves, relieve epilepsy (heart, liver);
>
> sea lion genitalia: salty, increase yang, sexual potency (aphrodisiac).

The most popular animal for medical purposes is the tiger. Many of its parts are used medicinally, so that one tiger may create $100,000 in revenue. Its bones are the most potent. Said to have a bitter taste, they are believed efficacious in expelling wind, stabilizing the nervous system, relieving pain, and alleviating epilepsy. Its pupils, moreover, help with anxiety and cramps; its brain is good for pimples; its teeth for asthma, rabies, and penile injuries; its gallbladder for digestive disorders; its stomach for stomach issues; its testicles for tuberculosis; its penis for enhancing the libido; its claws to strengthen *qi*; its fat for hemorrhoids and head injuries; its skin for mental disorders; and its tail for skin diseases (Alther, "Artenschutzrelevanz").

This popularity takes its toll. Three species of tigers are already extinct, and among the remaining two types only a few thousand survive. Similarly, rhinoceros in Africa have been reduced by 90 percent since the 1970s, and other animals, especially turtles and tortoises, are seriously affected. Another aspect of the animal ingredients in Chinese pharmaceuticals is cruelty to animals. For example, collar bears are raised in tiny cages for the production of gall fluid—about 15,000 pounds annually, used in medications against infections, cancer, hepatitis, hemorrhoids, digestive problems, and asthma. Other bears are not excluded: even

American grizzlies and black bears are being killed for their gallbladders. Legislation is in place, but implementation and enforcement lag.

> **Exercise:** How do you feel about the use of animals in medicine? About animal trials? If the animal is not threatened by extinction, does that make it okay? What do you think could and should be done to balance the needs of animals and the human demand for potent remedies and better drugs?

Above and beyond individual herbs and drug compounds, the highest form of Chinese *materia medica* are substances that not only enhance health and vitality but also aid the body in the transformation of *qi* into subtler and more spiritual forms, thus leading to long life and immortality. Daoist practitioners have experimented widely with herbal and other formulas and have created intricate elixirs for the attainment of spiritual goals. The *Immortals Biographies* (*Liexian zhuan*) of the Han dynasty mentions numerous medicines, including plants (cinnamon, peach, citrus peel, chrysanthemum flowers, calamus, pine, cedar, sesame, angelica, persimmons, lotus root, and mushrooms), animals (turtle shell, deer antlers), and minerals (mica, hematite, aconite, saltpeter, mercury, and cinnabar). The most popular is the pine tree, many parts of which are used, such as seeds, nuts, resin, bark, and roots.

Daoist religious literature contains many recipes for potent elixirs, often including common herbs. Their preparation is guided by the calendar and has to match astrological signs and seasonal cycles. They are often boiled, fried, and steamed, then buried for a period for greater enhancement. Their effects are tremendous. As the *Explanation of the Five Talismans* (*Wufuxu*), a religious manual of the fourth century C.E., says about a formula based on chrysanthemum flowers:

> Take it three times daily after meals. Within one year, all your ailments will disappear, your hearing will be sharp, your vision keen, your body light, your *qi* strong, and you will live long. After two years, your facial complexion will be joyful and glossy, your *qi* and vigor will multiply a hundredfold, white hairs will revert to black, and lost teeth will start to grow anew. You will live even longer.

> After three years, when you enter the mountains, you will no longer be in danger from snakes or dragons, sprites and demons will stay away from you, soldiers and armed robbers will be awed, and even the flying birds will show their respect. You will live for an extremely long time. (ch. 2)

The most potent of all Daoist immortality medicines were so-called cinnabar elixirs (*dan*). Based on both ordinary and rare ingredients—pine needles, pine resin, mushrooms, persimmons, apricot kernels, deer antlers, mother-of-pearl, mica, aconite, realgar, sulfur, mercury, arsenic, silver, and gold—their preparation required secrecy, ritual purification, and extended periods of time. As described in the *Book of the Master Who Embraces Simplicity* (*Baopuzi*, trl. Ware 1966) by the aristocrat Ge Hong (287–347), alchemists had to set up their furnace in a secluded spot with the right kind of *qi*, then time their work according to a cosmic schedule, observing the right times of firing and cooling, stirring and burying.

The process was thought to imitate the growth of gold in the earth on a microcosmic scale, and accordingly followed the stages of cosmic creation as it was perceived at the time. Essentially the work of the alchemist occurred on three levels: the concrete concoction of the elixir for immortality; the creation of gold from base metals for personal wealth; and the replication of the cosmic processes of creation for insights into, and power over, the innermost secrets of the universe. Alchemy was, therefore, both a chemical and a mystical endeavor which led not only to chemically induced trances and visions but also to the high spiritual states necessary for immortal transformation.

If and when the elixir had been created successfully, the alchemist had to perform a sacrifice of gratitude and give away large portions of the newly created gold to the gods and, anonymously, to the crowds. He could then take varying doses of the elixir, a gray-brown mud that was ingested either rolled into a pill or dissolved in liquid. Depending on the dose, he would attain various levels of magical powers, gain extensive divine protection, find a new level of lightness and radiance in body and mind, and have the choice of either extending his sojourn on earth indefinitely or ascending to heaven in broad daylight (Pregadio, "Elixirs").

As is obvious from the complexity of the undertaking, very few people managed to actually brew an elixir, and even if they did it often resulted in brain damage or death, interpreted as an increasing openness toward heavenly visions or the successful transformation into an immortal. Still, not only alchemists but also officials and even emperors undertook the quest, resulting in a number of untimely deaths. As a result, and especially when several emperors died from elixir poisoning in the Tang dynasty, operative alchemy was outlawed and serious practitioners turned toward the internal ingredients in the body, developing a new Daoist practice called inner alchemy which has survived to the present day.

Further Readings

Alther, Sandra. 2001. "Artenschutzrelevanz der Verwendung von Wildtieren in der traditionellen chinesischen Medizin." *Chinesische Medizin* 4/2001: 143-51.

Elias, Jason, and Katherine Ketcham. 1998. *The Five Elements of Self-Healing: Using Chinese Medicine for Maximum Immunity, Wellness, and Health.* New York: Harmony Books.

Fang, Chunyang. 2000. "Die Anwendung von Rettich in der chinesischen Diätetik." *Chinesische Medizin* 4/2000: 142-44.

Fulder, Stephen. 1993. *The Book of Ginseng and Other Chinese Herbs for Vitality.* Rochester, VT: Healing Arts Press.

Halpern, Georges. 1996. *Gingko: A Practical Guide.* New York: Avery Publishing Group.

Holmes, Peter. 1989. *The Energetics of Western Herbs: Treatment Strategies Integrating Western and Oriental Herbal Medicine.* 2 vols. Boulder: Snow Lion Press.

Mitchell, Craig, Feng Ye and Nigel Wiseman. 1999. *Shang Han Lun: On Cold Damage.* Brookline, Mass.: Paradigm Publications.

Pregadio, Fabrizio. 2000. "Elixirs and Alchemy." In *Daoism Handbook,* edited by Livia Kohn, 165-95. Leiden: E. Brill.

Rister, Robert. 1999. *Japanese Herbal Medicine: The Healing Art of Kampo.* Garden City Park, NY: Avery Publishing Group.

Stuart, G. A. 1976. *Chinese Materia Medica.* Taipei: Southern Materials Center.

Teeguarden, Ron. 1995. *Chinese Tonic Herbs.* New York: Japan Publications.

Ware, James R. 1966. *Alchemy, Medicine and Religion in the China of AD 320.* Cambridge, Mass.: MIT Press.

Chapter 15

Sexual Practices

Sexual energy is one of the major forms of *qi* in the human body. Defined as the visible and tangible form of *jing*, it resembles breath and food in its exchange with the outside world and role in maintaining health. Sexual energy emerges from the body's primordial *qi*, present in people from birth in limited amounts. Located in the Ocean of *Qi* (Qihai, CV-6, abdomen) in men and in the Cavern of *Qi* (Qixue, CV-17, chest) in women, *jing* transforms and assembles in the kidneys, more precisely in the glands located above them, the hormonal centers of the suprarenal glands or adrenal cortex of biomedicine.

Jing has varying effects on the body over a lifetime. In children it governs growth and maturation. During puberty, it arises more strongly and leads to sexual maturity: girls begin to menstruate and boys have first ejaculations. *Jing* reaches its peak in early adulthood when most people marry and have children. Then, with continued menstruation and ejaculation, it is increasingly lost until it diminishes to a trickle and stops completely—women reaching menopause, men no longer able to sustain an erection. Old age begins, with the classical indicators of white hair, loss of teeth, overall weakness, and various ailments—all symptoms associated with the decline of *jing* (Reid, *Tao of Health*, 294-97).

The key to the understanding of *jing* in Chinese medicine and Daoism is that its presence means life, vitality, and good health, while its absence is a harbinger of death, decline, and disease. It is also important to realize that the inborn store of *qi* which is periodically transformed into *jing* and then appears as sexual energy is limited and that every time a woman menstruates and a man ejaculates, valuable *qi* is lost, while health and life expectancy diminish. Whenever *jing* is lost through sexual activity, the brain, the bones of the head, and the skeleton of the body are weakened and become more brittle. Many diseases have accordingly been linked with the loss of sexual energy, from general weakness and dizziness, inability to concentrate, susceptibility to colds and infections to major problems, such as tuberculosis, anemia, osteoporosis, and kidney failure.

Vice versa, sexual dysfunction in Chinese medicine is associated with a lack of *jing* due to other activities, be it frequent masturbation, overexertion of the brain (injurious to heart and spleen), emotional strain leading to *qi*-stagnation, or dysfunction of the liver and kidneys caused by the downward drive of pathogenic damp-heat. Treatment focuses particularly on the kidneys, the main seat of *jing* after its transformation from *qi* and the organ associated with fear and anxiety, often named as causes of erectile dysfunction in the West.

Chinese therapy applies either the productive or the control cycle of the five phases. According to the productive cycle, water nourishes wood and if the kidneys fail, liver deficiency arises, creating symptoms of dizziness, blurred vision, headaches, muscle weakness, or spasms. According to the control cycle, water regulates fire, and if water fails to control fire, either excess or deficiency in the heart results—linking emotional turbulence with lack of *jing*. It also recommends certain dietary measures, encouraging sufferers to eat more carrots, bananas, pumpkin seeds, oysters, wheat germ oil, lecithin, and bee pollen.

As *jing* is the key to vitality and health and easily diminishes through sexual engagements, Chinese medicine and Daoism both focus on two issues: how to conserve the stock people have originally and how to replenish what is lost (or even to create more). The first—conservation—tends to focus on times and frequencies of intercourse as well as on massage techniques that keep the *qi* flowing. It does not advise celibacy, since the flow of sexual energy is important for health, and complete abstinence creates *qi*-blockages that do more harm than good in the long run. The second—replenishing—concentrates on the "return" or "reversion" of semen or menstrual blood into primordial *qi* with the help of both partner and solo practices.

Within this general framework, sexual practices occur on three levels, reflecting different intentions or mind-sets: (1) among ordinary people they are part of marital intercourse and focus largely on healing and conservation; (2) among longevity seekers they are known as "reverting sexual energy to nourish the brain" (*huanjing bunao*); they can be undertaken individually through meditative refinement or involve active intercourse, sometimes with multiple partners who are brought to orgasm while the practitioner retains *qi*; (3) and in organized Daoism sexual practices are known as "harmonization of *qi*" (*heqi*) among the early Celestial Masters and as "twosome cultivation" (*shuangxiu*) in the inner alchemy of late imperial China. Ritually transformed ways of intercourse, these techniques are employed to enhance oneness with the Dao and often lead on to solo practice, where yin and yang are isolated within the body and refined in an energetic and increasingly spiritual union.

Ordinary people who wish to maintain their health and vitality should be careful to manage their loss of *jing*. Men should learn not to experience full release in every sexual encounter and limit their ejaculations according to age. Younger men should have two or three ejaculations in every ten encounters, a number that goes down to one in twenty, thirty, fifty, or even a hundred as they get older. Men know that they are not overtaxing themselves if the sexual release leaves them light and refreshed, active and not sleepy. If they find themselves exhausted after climax, they should ejaculate less frequently. Women should ensure that menstruation is regular and neither too much nor too little. A certain regular release of blood is advisable for uterine health and physical harmony, just as ejaculations at regular intervals are important for men.

To stabilize sexual energy, both should practice the "deer exercise," a form of sexual massage, undertaken daily. Sit cross-legged, women pressing one heel against the perineum at the base of the pelvis, men cupping their testicles in one hand. Rub the hands together to get the *qi* moving, then massage the *qi*-center in the body in circular motion— women using both hands to gently rub over the breasts, men using the free hand to rub over the abdomen. Men change hands after eighty-one rounds and repeat. Women change direction after thirty-six rounds. Afterwards, with hands resting in the lap, practitioners of both sexes focus their attention inward to get a sense of soft sexual energy flowing through the body. To conclude, they contract the perineum muscles, hold them tight while continuing to breathe, then release. It is common to feel a warm, sexual glow rise through the body, the tangible presence of *jing* (Cohen, *Way of Qigong*, 320).

> **Exercise:** Reflect on your personal perception of sexual energy. Do you see it as unlimited, threatening, pleasurable, a source of power, a basis for health, or what? How is your perception different from the Chinese? How does it reflect Western cultural values?

Sexual exchange with a loving partner should be undertaken regularly. However, there are certain times when it is not recommended to have sex: after a heavy meal, when intoxicated, after strenuous activity or an acupuncture treatment, when acutely ill, during emotional upheaval, when suffering pressure in the bladder or bowels, during menstruation, and at times of severe, inclement weather. All of these are situations that upset the internal *qi* balance of the person. They need to be resolved before successful sexual activity can be experienced. In the *Secret Recipes from a Jade Chamber* (*Yufang bijue*), the Master of Pure Harmony (Chonghezi) points out some more details:

> If you have sex at midnight, before you have fully digested your evening meal, you may develop chest pain and fullness of *qi*. Indications are a pulling sensation beneath the ribs and pressure in the breast, as if it were being torn. You will lose your appetite for food and drink, feel a blocking knot beneath your heart, sometimes even vomit green and yellow bile. Your stomach will feel tense with the fullness of energy and there will be a slow and irregular pulse. Sometimes in addition there may be nosebleeds, hardness or pain beneath the ribs, and sores on the face. To heal this, have intercourse after midnight and close to the approach of dawn. . . .
>
> To cure this by means of sexual techniques, rise at cockcrow and use the bathroom. Then return to your bed, settle yourself comfortably and slowly engage in playful dalliance. When your entire body is deeply relaxed, cause your partner to be slippery with secretions, then withdraw. The illness will be wonderfully cured. The same method also helps in female maladies. (Wile, *Arts of the Bedchamber*, 103)

To enhance sexual enjoyment, partners should take certain herbs and teas, such as ginseng, cinnamon, cardamom, nutmeg, ginger, and other warming, yang-inducing substances. Before engaging in sexual activity, they should create a pleasant atmosphere in a clean environment and prepare by taking a bath. It is good to allow plenty of time for foreplay, making sure both partners are ready and aroused, focusing on the exchange of *qi* in mouth, breasts, and genitals—stimulating the jade spring (saliva), the white snow (nipple *qi*), and the moon flower (vaginal excretion). Both male and female sexual secretions contain hormones, enzymes, proteins, and vitamins, and both benefit from their exchange.

As practitioners engage in frequent sucking and kissing, they gradually attain readiness for intercourse. In the male, relevant signs are elongation, swelling, hardness, and heat, aided by a massage of feet and toes which contain meridian endings and support sexual vitality. In women, signs include a flushed face, hardened nipples, a "parched throat, dry lips, and difficulty swallowing," followed by wetness in the jade gate, and a thick fluid flowing down the thighs (Reid, *Tao of Health*, 269).

Once both partners are engaged, the male has a variety of thrusting styles: left and right, under and over, in and out, deep and shallow, deep and fast, rise and plunge, slow and push, fast and poised. Each thrust, moreover, can be executed at various levels, be it shallow, medium, deep, or very deep. Longer and more frequent thrusting is said to be good for health, and many diseases are cured by practicing eighty-one strokes nine times daily, for a period of nine days.

Variety is the spice of good sex. Couples are encouraged to experiment with various positions, including the turning dragon, stalking tiger, leaping monkey, mating cicada, mounting tortoise, fluttering phoenix, sucking rabbit, overlapping fish scales, and cranes joining neck:, all geared to increase potency, sexual enjoyment, and overall health (Reid, *Tao of Health*, 318-25).

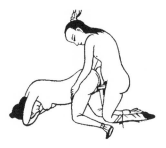

Fig. 28. The stalking tiger.

When they reach climax, *qi* is exchanged in a powerful burst that is enhanced by a few well advised measures:

> Keep your head nuzzled under your partner's ear when he or she ejaculates in order to avoid inhaling the 'muddy breath' exhaled at that moment. Owing to the intense 'fire' that occurs in the lower abdomen during orgasm, this burst of breath is regarded as a sort of waste product.

> Hug your partner very tightly and maintain maximum surface contact between your skins. At orgasm, the entire body radiates energy from its surface contact. Press and rub the pubic regions very closely together. The biggest burst of sexual energy during orgasm naturally occurs in the region of the Ocean of *Qi*, located below the navel. (Reid, *Tao of Health*, 291)

For these practices, ideally intercourse should take place between consenting adults of different sexes. Homosexuality, although present in traditional China and reported variously in historical records, is not mentioned in Chinese medical texts, which tend to support the active exchange between yin and yang and the traditional Chinese family structure. Thus they reformulate the five Confucian virtues in a sexual context, emphasizing that partners should practice benevolence by approaching sex with generosity; righteousness by having intercourse at appropriate times; propriety by showing mutual respect and restraint; reciprocity by keeping an open attitude about the other's weaknesses; and wisdom by knowing themselves and learning about each other. Altogether, regular, well-measured and mutually enjoyable sex among committed partners has many benefits. It aids the concentration of *jing*, rests the spirit, benefits the organs, strengthens the bones, harmonizes blood circulation, increases the blood, balances the five phases, and in general helps to adjust the entire system.

> **Exercise:** Reflect on the medical understanding of sex in Western culture. Is it considered helpful or harmful? How do psychological attitudes influence it?

In longevity practice and for healing, sexual practice is modified further. First there are a number of sexual techniques that can be used to improve eyesight, hearing, and other bodily functions. The Master of Pure Harmony says:

> To improve your eyesight, wait for the impulse to ejaculate, then raise your head, hold the breath, and expel the air with a loud sound, while rolling your eyes to the left and right. Contract your abdomen and revert the *jing* upward so that it enters the hundred vessels of the body. . . .

> To improve the functioning of your five organs, facilitate digestion, and cure the hundred ills, wait for the approach of ejaculation, then expand your belly and mentally move the *qi* around the body. Next, contract your belly again so that the *jing* disperses and reverts to the hundred vessels. Then penetrate your partner nine times shallow and once deeply between her zither strings and grain ears. Good *qi* will return, ill *qi* will depart. (Wile, *Arts*, 104)

Most technical instructions such as these are directed at men who are to create a state of arousal in a sexual encounter, wait for the urge to ejaculate, then—holding their breath, clenching their teeth, and contracting the perineum muscles—prevent ejaculation and instead guide the aroused *jing* back into the body, moving it up along the spine and circulating it through the torso. This method is "reverting the sexual energy to nourish the brain."

This practice stands at the center of sexual longevity techniques known as "bedchamber arts" (*fangzhong shu*), documented first in the Mawangdui manuscripts of 168 B.C.E. Since then they have been written up in various manuals, commonly associated with female masters instructing the Yellow Emperor, such as the Simple Woman (Sunü), the Colorful Woman (Cainü), and the Mysterious Woman (Xuannü).

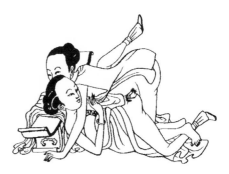

Fig. 29. Therapeutic love posture for strengthening the bones.

Often these works became "pillow books," that is, texts rolled up in hollow neck supports made from bamboo, wood, or porcelain. Sexual instructions were also recorded in general books on longevity and make up an entire chapter in the Japanese encyclopedia *Essential Medical Methods* (ch. 28), which forms the basis for most English presentations.

The bedchamber arts taught men to have interrupted intercourse, ideally with as many women as possible, preferably young and healthy ones. They should bring their partners to orgasm so the women would emit their sexual essence but never have an ejaculation themselves. The doctrine behind the practices assumes that while women's *qi* is lost through transformation into menstrual blood they possess an inexhaustible supply of yin fluids and will not suffer from having frequent orgasms. On the other hand, it also assumes that the women will not easily agree to be used by men, and the literature describes the practices as a battle. For example, a passage from the *Prayer Mat of the Flesh* (*Roubu duan*), a sixteenth-century novel with numerous sex scenes, states:

> Apart from the number of combatants involved, are there really any differences between battles fought by armies and those fought in bed? In both cases, the commanders' first priority is to survey the terrain and assess the opponent. In sexual encounters, it is the hills and valleys of the woman that first attract the man's attention, while she is most curious about the size and firepower of his weapons. Who will advance and who

> will retreat? In bed as in war, it is just as important to know
> yourself as it is to know your opponent. (Reid, *Tao*, 266)

Beyond the male mainstream, some documents also encourage women
to take similar advantage of male partners. The most prominent model
for this behavior is the Queen Mother of the West (Xiwang mu), a major
Daoist goddess who successfully gained long life through sexual intercourse with men. Based on her model, the Master of Pure Harmony has
appropriate advice for women:

> When having intercourse with a man, first calm your heart and
> still your mind. If the man is not yet fully aroused, wait for his
> *qi* to arrive and restrain your emotions in order to attune your-
> self to him. Do not move or become agitated, lest your yin es-
> sence become exhausted first. If this happens, you will be left
> in a deficient state and be susceptible to illnesses due to wind
> and cold. . . .
>
> If you do not have intercourse for the sake of offspring, you
> can divert the fluids to flow back into the hundred vessels of
> your body. By using yang to nourish yin, the various ailments
> disappear, your complexion becomes radiant and your flesh
> strong. Then you can enjoy long life without aging and be
> young forever. (Wile, *Arts*, 103)

On a third level, sexual practices also played a role in religious Daoism
which both rejected and embraced them in different contexts. The organized groups of the second century C.E., the Way of Great Peace (Taiping
dao) and the Celestial Masters (Tianshi), sublimated sexual partner practices in ritual intercourse. With their strong millenarian belief systems,
ritually based hierarchies, moral lifestyle, and intense community cohe-
sion, these groups formed the backbone of the organized Daoist religion.
They understood sexuality as the most direct and most obvious way of
harmonizing and integrating yin and yang, leading to a state of unitary
qi and thus to harmony with the Dao. They did not favor either sex, but
allotted a specific role to each partner: the yang creating and engender-
ing, the yin transforming and transmuting.

In ritual intercourse early Daoists learned to detach themselves from desire and dissociate orgasm from pleasure. The act itself was less important than its effect of setting the *qi* in harmonious motion along the bodily circuits, where it provided sustenance and nourishment. Daoists pri-
oritized the internal over the external, the invisible over the visible, in

order to allow full empowerment of the harmony of the two forces, thereby benefiting themselves, their community, and the cosmos at large.

Exercise: Reflect on the role of sexuality in religion and on the different attitudes religions have exhibited toward sexuality in human history. Are there other traditions that have made use of sexual forces for religious attainment? What other attitudes have there been and with what justification?

Members of the Way of Great Peace and the Celestial Masters, underwent initiatory rites known as the harmonization of *qi*, during which male sexual energies (yellow *qi*) and female sexual energies (red *qi*) joined together in accord with cosmic forces. Assembling in the oratory before a master, adepts began with slow, formal movements accompanied by meditations to create a sacred space, then established the harmony between their *qi* and the cosmic *qi* through visualizations. As described in a medieval Daoist text:

> May each person visualize the *qi* of his cinnabar field as large as a six-inch mirror, leaving the body through open space. Its light progressively increases to illuminate the head and bathe the entire body in radiance, so that the adept can clearly discern the five inner organs, the six viscera, the nine palaces, the twelve lodgings, the four limbs, as well as all the joints, vessels, pores, and defensive and nutritive *qi* within the body and without. (Despeux and Kohn, *Women in Daoism*, 12)

Next, adepts informed the master and the gods that they were going to undertake the harmonization of *qi*. This involved sexual intercourse guided by ritualistic movements in precise directions and according to astronomically defined positions. During the act practitioners strove for the maintenance of bodily essence and vital spirits through the retention of sexual fluids. Reverting the fluids away from orgasmic expulsion, practitioners would move them up along the spinal column and into the head, where they supposedly nourished the brain and enhanced the individual's health and the community's harmony. The risen *qi* would also communicate with the gods of the heavens who erased the names of all participating members from the registers of death and inscribed them in the ledgers of immortality.

The other major form of Daoist partner practice arose in late imperial China as part of inner alchemy. Called "twosome cultivation" and still used in inner alchemy today, it serves as an initial stage in the preparation for the advanced creation of an internal elixir of immortality. Undertaken with specially trained women in a sacred chamber — with numerous rooms and altars dedicated to various deities and lineage masters — the ritual intercourse begins with purification, then proceeds through formal worship and incantations to a carefully orchestrated joining of mutual energetic forces. It tames sexual instincts and allows practitioners to expand sexual energies into cosmic qi. Eventually the partners can exchange sexual energies without even touching. Their energy fields merge in an explosive, all-embracing orgasm, moving both outward as their spirits travel into the planetary vastness of the otherworld and inward as the body is opened to cosmic emptiness and primordiality. The experience is overwhelming and transcendent, yet firmly grounded in the energetics of the body, activated with a partner, yet ultimately a transformation of the individual (Winn, "Spiritual Orgasm"). The cosmic oneness it affords can, moreover, also be reached by alchemically transmuting sexual energy in solo practice — described in chapter 20 below.

Further Readings

Abrams, Douglas, and Mantak Chia. 2000. *The Multi-Orgasmic Couple: Sexual Secrets Every Couple Should Know*. San Francisco: Harper San Francisco.

Chia, Mantak, and Michael Winn. 1984. *Taoist Secrets of Love: Cultivating Male Sexual Energy*. Santa Fe: Aurora Press.

Chu, Valentin. 1993. *The Yin-Yang Butterfly*. New York: Putnam.

Despeux, Catherine, and Livia Kohn. 2003. *Women in Daoism*. Cambridge, Mass.: Three Pines Press.

Foucault, Michel. 1986. *The History of Sexuality. Volume Three: The Care of the Self*. New York: Pantheon Books.

Gulik, Robert H. van. 1961. *Sexual Life in Ancient China*. Leiden: E. Brill.

Reid, Daniel P. 1989. *The Tao of Health, Sex, and Longevity*. New York: Simon & Schuster.

Wile, Douglas. 1992. *Art of the Bedchamber: The Chinese Sexology Classics*. Albany: State University of New York Press.

Winn, Michael. 2002. "The Quest for Spiritual Orgasm: Daoist and Tantric Sexual Cultivation in the West." www.healingdao.com/cgi-bin/articles.pl

Chapter 16
Breathing and Gymnastics

Above and beyond clinical healing and interactive *qi*-control, Chinese health methods also include various techniques of self-cultivation. Undertaken individually under the guidance of a master, they are set in a religious and spiritual context and do not primarily aim at healing. Still, they often also have a medicinal effect on body and mind. Breathing exercises are a major way of self-cultivation. They serve to control *qi* and ensure health, longevity, and a greater sense of alignment with the Dao. Also an important part of Ayurveda and Yoga, where they are known as *pranayâma* (e.g., Farhi, *Breathing Book*), breath control goes back far in history. In China it is first mentioned in the *Book of Master Zhuang* and in Han-dynasty manuscripts. These texts describe breathing as essential for good health and therefore for long life and the pursuit of religious goals.

In Western science, too, numerous studies acknowledge the connection of breath to health (e.g., Loehr, *Breathe In*; www.authentic-breathing.com). As they show, when people are stressed, their breathing becomes shallow and short, and before long they accept this as normal. They adapt to no longer using the deeper part of the lungs, where the blood flow rate is faster and the renewal of energy greatest, thus depriving themselves of a great source of vigor and renewal.

Breathing only as deep as the chest has several effects on the body. For one, it necessitates the taking of more breaths, so that instead of 10 to12 deep and relaxed breaths per minute, stressed people take 16 or more. This causes the heart to beat faster and work overtime, making it wear out that much sooner. Heart disease and cardio-pulmonary conditions are the eventual result. Also, breathing in a stressful manner prevents sufficient amounts of oxygen from reaching the cells. Instead of exchanging fresh oxygen for old carbon dioxide in the lungs and thereby giving new energy to their system, stressed people take in oxygen only in very small quantities and maintain an unhealthy amount of gaseous toxins in the body. This in turn causes the blood to become more acidic and tension to build up. The hypothalamus and pituitary glands are stimulated, stress hormones such as cortisol and adrenaline are released, and they in turn fuel the sense of urgency, tension, and anxiety. Breathing becomes even shallower and more rapid, leading to a vicious circle that ends in decline, sickness, and early death (www.breathware.com; www.breathmastery. com; www. breathttherapy.net).

> **Exercise:** Over a day or two, make an effort to note your own breathing pattern. How is your breathing when you get up in the morning? When you are on your way to class/work? When you face a problem? When you eat? When you have fun? And so on. Overall, what is your dominant tendency in breathing?

The Chinese have been aware of the power of breath for a long time. Their most general term for breathing exercises is "expelling the old and taking in the new" (*tugu naxin*). This describes breathing in deeply and abdominally through the nose ("gate of heaven") and exhaling through the mouth ("doorway of earth"). Doing so, people inhale fresh, vital *qi* while expelling its impure, gross counterpart.

This, or any other form of breathing practice, should be done in a clean, tranquil setting while avoiding all foulness and defilement. As *Master Taiwu's Qi Scripture* (*Taiwu xiansheng qijing*) says:

> Whenever you are nourishing, refining, or ingesting *qi*, avoid foulness by staying away from births and funerals. Do not smell the bad miasma of dead cattle or anything else that is rotten, unclean, impure, and the like. If you see something ominous, stinking, or unclean, you must chant an incantation to rid yourself of the defilement. Otherwise your proper *qi* will be harmed. (Huang and Wurmbrand, *Primordial Breath*, 29)

Having made sure of the proper setting and cleanliness, adepts prepare by reducing their food intake, since over-consumption taxes the system and lower amounts allow the energies to circulate freely. They then undertake various forms of breathing practice, commonly beginning with two basic methods: enclosing the *qi* (*biqi*), and guiding the *qi* (*xingqi*).

Enclosing the *qi* is a form of holding the breath. It is best done at the time of rising yang, between midnight and noon, in a high, dry, quiet, and secluded room. Adepts burn incense and lie down on a bed that is raised well above the ground to prevent earth-*qi* from impacting the practice. They rest on their backs and support their necks on a pillow. Then they close the eyes, curl the hands into fists—so that no *qi* can escape—inhale deeply, and hold the breath. The *Record on Nurturing Inner Nature and Extending Life* (*Yangxing yanming lu*), a seventh-century manual on longevity techniques, says:

Lie down straight, close your eyes, and curl your hands into fists [the four fingers covering the thumb]. Enclose the *qi* and do not breathe. Mentally count to 200, then expel the *qi* by exhaling through the mouth. As you breathe like this for an increasing number of days, you will find your body, spirit, and all the five organs at peace.

If you can enclose the *qi* to the count of 250, your Flowery Canopy [lungs] will be radiant. Your eyes and ears will be perceptive and clear, and your body will be light and free from disease; nothing wayward will bother you. (ch. 2)

The first effect of holding the breath for a substantial period is that the body begins to sweat, which eliminates colds and other disorders through the skin—associated with the lungs and part of the body's breathing apparatus. In the long run, holding the breath also expands lung capacity and increases quietude of mind, since the body is brought to extreme stillness. It also helps with eliminating hunger and thirst.

The second basic method is guiding the *qi*. This is a mental exercise undertaken once the breath has entered the body. It is first mentioned in the late Zhou dynasty, when an inscription describes how adepts perform an initial downward movement of *qi*, followed by its transformation and upward return. The practice begins by inhaling through the nose and exhaling through the mouth. Gradually the breath becomes subtle and gets longer. Using this concentrated long breath, upon inhalation, practitioners let the *qi* settle in the lower cinnabar field. On exhalation, they see it move down to the pelvic floor. During the next inhalation, they feel it flow upward along the spine, reaching the shoulders and head. The following exhalation brings the *qi* over the head to the nostrils. This breath can be undertaken through the nostrils only or by breathing in through the nose and out through the mouth. The course of the *qi* follows the track of the Governing and Conception Vessels in the microcosmic orbit, part of Qigong exercises and Daoist meditation.

Guiding the *qi* is also used to heal specific ailments. As the *Record on Nurturing Inner Nature* says: "Guide the *qi* in order to expel the hundred illnesses. Follow it wherever it is needed and develop clear awareness there. If your head hurts, become aware of your head; if your foot hurts, become aware of your foot, using harmonized *qi* to deal with the pain. From one moment to the next, it will dissolve by itself" (ch. 2). This means that any specific ailment in the body can be relieved and even cured through the conscious guiding of *qi* to the problem area. *Qi* is used as a means to open the body and to allow the congestion to dissolve, thus eliminating pain and discomfort.

> **Exercise:** Go to the web and look up modern ways of using breath to relieve various health conditions. Look for "transformational breathing," "rebirthing," and the like.

A more complex breathing method involves "ingesting *qi*" (*shiqi*), also known as "swallowing *qi*" (*yinqi*). Its goal is to replace food intake with *qi*, thus sublimating the body. To do this, adepts sit in a meditative posture, either kneeling or cross-legged, with the back and neck straight, the eyes closed, and the mind concentrated. They take in *qi* through the nose and hold it in the mouth to mix it with saliva—a potent form of *qi* known as "jade spring" or "sweet wine."

Using the mix of saliva and breath, adepts rinse the mouth and gain a feeling of fullness, allowing the *qi* to envelope the tongue and teeth. Then they consciously swallow it, visualizing the mixture as it moves into the torso and to the inner organs. Once the *qi* is safely stored in its intended receptacle, they exhale. In the long run, this has a strong effect. As the *Record on Nurturing Inner Nature* says, "If you can do one thousand swallowings like this in one day and night, this is most excellent." Swallowing and ingesting *qi* over longer periods, thereby accessing the *qi* of the seasons and at different times of day, eventually makes the abdomen feel full and eliminates the need for food and drink.

Qi-ingestion is a preparation for *bigu*, the "abstention from grains." To modify their diet, practitioners begin by taking simpler foods, such as rice porridge, boiled wheat dumplings, cooked barley, and dried meat, as well as raw pepper corns to make the *qi* harmonious and to ward off cold, heat, and dampness. After a few weeks of deep breathing and this simple diet, they can start skipping one or two meals. They replace grains with steamed vegetables, seasoned with soy sauce or vinegar and enhanced with medicinal herbs. This cleanses the colon and weans the body from its need for grains. After another week, adepts can do away with the vegetables, too, taking only their juice. Three days later, food intake ceases but liquids should still be taken as well as a few daily pepper corns (Huang and Wurmbrand, *Primordial Breath*, 60).

While the methods of enclosing and guiding the *qi* use the lungs and skin as their main route of healing, the ingesting and swallowing *qi* impacts most on the digestive system, emptying the stomach, cleansing the intestines, and thereby releasing toxins and wayward *qi*. A wider range of effects is found in yet a different practice that refines the main organs: known as the Six Breaths (*liuqi fa*), it involves inhaling deeply while visualizing an organ and its color, then exhaling from the organ in a specific manner. For example, *si* is the breath of the lungs, a gentle, relaxed exhalation that lets the breath escape between slightly opened lips. "If you feel blocking heat, disharmony, or exhaustion, use this breath. Or again, if your skin is ulcerated, painful, or swollen, rely on this breathing method and the condition will clear up" (*Primordial Breath*, 24).

Similarly, the breath of the heart is *he*. It is a strong breath with open mouth, accompanied by a guttural rasping through tightening of the throat. It helps in cases of dry tongue and congestion or tension in the chest. For the spleen and conditions associated with the stomach, use the *hu* breath, blowing it out with rounded lips; for the liver and problems with the eyes, use *xu*, a gentle expulsion with open mouth; and for the kidneys and diseases of ears, genitals, and legs, use *chui*, a sharp expulsion of air, with lips almost closed. The sixth sound is *xi* and associated with the triple heater. Traditionally the sound of sighing, it is a soft exhalation with the mouth slightly open, used to balance all internal processes (Despeux, "Six Breaths").

While the Six Breaths harmonize the organs, a more spiritual practice known as the Five Sprouts (*wuya*) connects people with the five phases. The sprouts are the germinal essences of the five directions and represent the yin principle of heaven. Tender like fresh sprouts of plants, they assemble at dawn in the celestial capital, then spread all over the universe until the sun rises. Turning like the wheels of a carriage, they ascend to the gates of the Nine Heavens, from where they continue to the five sacred mountains on earth and eventually descend into the individual adept. Adepts ingest the Five Sprouts at dawn after lighting incense. They visualize the stars protecting them, and begin by inhaling *qi* and swallowing saliva. They then visualize the *qi* of each direction in its appropriate color and allow it to coalesce into a pill, which they swallow and guide to its matching organ (Robinet, *Taoist Meditation*).

Exercise: Sit down facing east. Imagine a green hue of mist or fog in front of you. Concentrate and allow the green hue to become denser until it forms into a ball. Shrink it mentally until it is just a small pill. Guide it towards your mouth and allow it to enter. Feel it move through your mouth, throat, and lungs into the liver. Envision the liver with a shining green hue of cosmic energy. How does this feel? Can you get a cosmic connection?

Another spiritual breathing practice is "embryo respiration" (*taixi*), i.e. breathing internally like the embryo in the womb. As Daoist adepts merge with the Dao, they can regulate and nurture the *qi* within, creating a closed world of energetic transformation. For this practice, they clap the teeth to announce the commencement of sacred activities, then roll their necks to loosen the *qi*-flow. They swallow the breath a number of times, mixing it with saliva as collected from the gums and teeth. Then they lie down, make their hands into fists, close the passes in and out of the body, and envision the *qi* nurturing their body within. Doing so, they create their own inner world by focusing their attention on the abdomen and concentrating on the *qi* moving in the torso. They envision it circulating as light, increasingly loosening their ties to the outer world and becoming more receptive to the Dao.

The modern version of these various breathing techniques developed through the work of Jiang Weiqiao (1870-1955) and is described in his *Quiet Sitting with Master Yinshi* (*Yinshizi jingzuo fa*; dat. 1914). Born in the 1870s, Jiang Weiqiao was a sickly child. In his teenage years he contracted TB and became increasingly unable to lead a normal life, but neither Western nor Chinese medicine could help him. His condition only improved when he found a text on Daoist techniques and started to follow its instructions. Within a year, a strict regimen of gymnastics, breathing, walks, meditations, and specific diets, restored not only his health but brought him to new spiritual dimensions (Lu, *Secrets*).

In *Quiet Sitting*, he distinguishes natural, deep, abdominal breathing, which should be used at all times, from regulated or reversed breathing, for which the abdominal muscles are held tight and the side ribs and back are expanded. He recommends mastery over natural breathing before practicing the reversed method, because it can cause dizziness and shortness of breath. He also describes how the *qi* in his body began to take on a life of its own, flowing naturally into the microcosmic orbit and exiting through the top of his head, taking all his weaknesses and ailments with it. His successful healing and presentation of traditional practices in a modern language laid the foundation for the later development of Qigong (Kohn, "Quiet Sitting").

Breathing exercises also form an essential part of Chinese gymnastics, *daoyin* (Jap. *dôin*), literally "guide [the *qi*] and stretch [the body]." Prescribing gentle movements to regulate *qi*-flow and expel pathogenic elements, gymnastics are a valuable tool to prevent old age and to cure diseases. They nourish the *qi*, refresh the body after hard work, help fasting and other spiritual practices, and open the body for a joyful life (see www.daoyintao.com; www.daoyin.it).

Gymnastics have been popular since antiquity, as the *Gymnastics Chart* (*Daoyin tu*) documents. This chart, found in a Han tomb at Mawangdui, consists of a series of illustrated exercises with short captions. The practices have colorful names: bear hangings, bird stretchings, monkey leaps, owl glares, and so on. They were used in conjunction with self-massages to dissolve blockages, help circulation, and increase the harmony of *qi*.

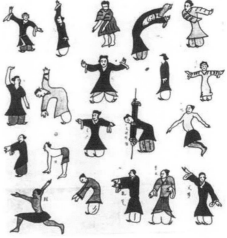

Fig. 30. Images from the *Gymnastics Chart*.

Another early manuscript, discovered at Zhangjia shan in Hunan and dated to 186 B.C.E., bears the title *Gymnastics Book* (*Yinshu*). It begins with the description of a daily and seasonal health regimen, then outlines over a hundred different exercises in three sections, some preventative, others more curative. In each case, it providing practice instructions, numbers of repetitions, and health benefits. A third part outlines briefly which technique is good for what ailment, as for example:

> Triple stretch is good for the shoulders.
> Tiger turn is good for the neck.
> Limbs dropping is good for the armpits.
> Turn and shake is good for abdomen and belly.
> (Engelhardt, "*Daoyin tu* und *Yinshu*")

Later, gymnastic methods were collected in integrated scriptures, most comprehensively in the *Gymnastics Classic* (*Daoyin jing*). It prescribes that gymnastic movements should be undertaken in a quiet setting, in a closed room rather than outdoors. One should have a mat or bed, ideally a raised platform that keeps the disruptive *qi* of the earth away. When one performs the exercises for therapy, the specific direction toward which they are aimed does not seem to matter. But when they are used as longevity techniques, there are some instructions on geographical orientation, with the east being the most common.

Gymnastic exercises can be divided into three types on the basis of posture, i.e., standing, sitting, and lying down Most of the early diagrams represent the standing style, commonly executed in parallel stance—standing straight with feet parallel and shoulder-width apart, knees relaxed and weight evenly distributed. But there are also practices undertaken in the horse stance (with knees bent further), single-foot stance (knees bent, weight on one foot), and bow stance (one leg forward and bent, the other back and straight). Moving patterns include both forward and backward moves, lifting the leg and putting the foot down in a controlled manner. In all these stances, the limbs and torso are rotated and stretched in accordance with regulated breathing. For example, Master Ning states:

> Stand parallel. Interlace your fingers above your head. Stretch up, then bend to the ground. Continue for five breaths. This fills the abdomen with energy.

> Stand on tiptoe. Hold your breath to the count of eight. This will free you from all ailments above the chest, i.e., those of the head, ears, eyes, throat, and nose.

> Make both hands into fists and clasp them to the back of your head. Hold your breath. Rise up on your toes. Hold your breath to the count of nine. Face east. This causes *qi* to move up and down, opens and deepens its passage through the nostrils, and cures all emaciation and weakness. (*Gymnastics Classic*, 3a)

Seated practice is usually undertaken in the cross-legged position. The back is straight, the head lifted, the weight evenly distributed. The joints of the body are moved gently and in the rhythm of the breath. For example, Master Redpine's instructions say:

> Fold your arms across your chest. Turn your head left and right. Hold your breath for as long as you can. This stretches the face and ear muscles. It expels wayward *qi* and prevents it from reentering the body.

> Now, link your hands behind your back as low as your buttocks. Turn your torso to the right and left as far as you can.

> Interlace your fingers in front of your body. Stretch your arms forward and turn them to the right and left as far as you can. This expands shoulder *qi*.

Next, interlace your fingers and stretch your arms above your head [with palms facing out]. Turn left and right in an easy rhythm. This expands the *qi* of the lungs and the liver. (1b)

Gymnastics undertaken while lying down include practices while on one's back or on one side. Another section of Master Redpine's instructions states:

Lie down on your right side and try to touch the ground to your left with your left elbow. Then stretch the left arm as much as you can and reach beyond your head. Repeat the exercise with your right arm while lying on your left side. Continue for five breaths. This stretches the muscles and the back.

Roll onto your back. Place both hands around your right knee and pull it up towards your waist and groin, raising your head at the same time to meet it. Repeat with the left knee. Continue for five breaths. This stretches the hips.

Place your right hand on your left knee, raised above your hip. Then stretch your left hand upward as far as you can. Repeat on the other side. Continue for five breaths. This expands the *qi* in chest and abdomen.

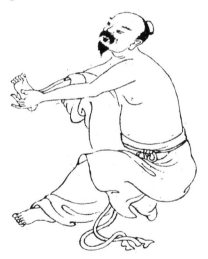

Place your left hand next to your hip and pull down. At the same time, stretch your right arm upward as far as you can. Repeat on the other side. Continue for five breaths. This expands the *qi* in the center of the body. (1ab)

Fig. 31. A summer exercise to supplement yin.

> **Exercise:** Try one or the other of the gymnastic sequences described. Do they work? How do they feel? Do they seem similar to modern exercises?

Over the years, specific sequences of gymnastic exercises developed, often associated with animals. An important set is the so-called Five Animals' Frolic (*wuqin xi*), associated with the physician Hua Tuo (141-203 C.E.) and including the crane, bear, deer, tiger, and monkey.

In the wake of Hua Tuo and under the influence of numerous later masters, Chinese gymnastics grew into a complex system of practices that involved a variety of moves and postures, with sequences often named after animals. Thus, the more recent *Illustrated Description of Inner and Outer Practices* (*Neiwai gong tushuo*) includes entire sequences of dragon and tiger moves, a collection of the methods of various famous immortals, and numerous practices to cure specific ailments (Berk, *Chinese Healing Arts*). In all cases, some moves are simple stretches that loosen up specific parts of the body and increase *qi* awareness; others involve extensive patterns of both movements and stretches. They have, to a large extent, been integrated into the Qigong movement today.

Further Readings

Berk, William R. 1986. *Chinese Healing Arts: Internal Kung-Fu*. Burbank, Calif.: Unique Publications.

Despeux, Catherine. 1989. "Gymnastics: The Ancient Tradition." In *Taoist Meditation and Longevity Techniques*, edited by Livia Kohn, 223-61. Ann Arbor: University of Michigan, Center for Chinese Studies Publications.

Despeux, Catherine. forthcoming. "The Six Breaths." In *Daoist Body Cultivation*, edited by Livia Kohn.

Engelhardt, Ute. 2001. "*Daoyin tu* und *Yinshu*: Neue Erkenntnisse über die Übungen zur Lebenspflege in der frühen Han-Zeit." *Monumenta Serica* 49: 213-26.

Farhi, Donna. 1996. *The Breathing Book*. New York: Henry Holt & Co.

Huang, Jane, and Michael Wurmbrand. 1987. *The Primordial Breath: Ancient Chinese Ways of Prolonging Life Through Breath*. Torrance, Calif.: Original Books.

Kohn, Livia. 2002. "Quiet Sitting with Master Yinshi: The Beginnings of Qigong in Modern China." In *Living With the Dao: Conceptual Issues in Daoist Practice*, edited by Livia Kohn, 140-55. Cambridge, Mass.: Three Pines Press.

Loehr, James E., and Jeffrey A. Migdow. 1986. *Breathe In, Breathe Out: Inhale Energy and Exhale Stress by Guiding and Controlling Your Breathing*. Alexandria, Virg.: Time Life Books.

Lu Kuan-yü. 1964. *The Secrets of Chinese Meditation*. London: Rider.

Robinet, Isabelle. 1993. *Taoist Meditation*. Translated by Norman Girardot and Julian Pas. Albany: State University of New York Press.

Chapter 17

Qigong

Qigong, usually rendered "Qi Exercises" but literally meaning the "effort" or the "merit" of *qi*, describes a group of practices highly popular in China and increasingly well known the West. Continuing the tradition of breathing and gymnastics, Qigong includes physical as well as meditation exercises, healing efforts, and (more recently) martial arts. What they all have in common is their activation and nourishing of *qi* in the human body through the application of specific techniques and thereby aiding it in the recovery of original health. People who practice Qigong regularly profess to attaining a state of strength and vigor, and many feel youthful even into hoary old age (www.qi.org; www.nqa.org).

Although Qigong continues many exercises that go back far in Chinese history, the term is quite recent and goes back to the 1940s. In 1947, the Communist Party cadre Liu Guizhen (1920-1983), suffering from a virulent gastric ulcer, was sent home to recover or die. He went home but refused to die—he was only 27 years old at the time! Instead, he took lessons in gymnastics and breathing from the Daoist Liu Duzhou. After 102 days of faithfully undertaking these practices, he was completely cured. He returned to his job and described his healing success to the Party, which appointed him as a medical research leader in Hebei province with the task to study the effects of breathing on healing. In 1948, he created the term *Qigong* to indicate the methods which focused largely on breathing at the time. He then began to teach Party officials and repeated his success with various ailments.

Qigong is undertaken in all postures of the body—standing, moving, sitting, and lying down. Always connected with deep, abdominal breathing and encouraging a state of inward absorption and relaxation, it consists for the most part of short exercises that are geared toward *qi*-activation and specific medical problems. As in traditional breathing practice, the mind in Qigong is used to visualize the *qi*-flow to specific areas in the body or its absorption from heaven and earth (Cohen, *Way of Qigong*, 129). The most common application of Qigong is self-applied in a series of daily practices, but it can also be activated through *qi*-infusion by a trained practitioner in a form of therapeutic touch or sent by a master over long distances by the mere power of thought.

Highly popular especially in the 1980s and 1990s, Qigong has grown to include many different techniques. It maintains several of the traditional breathing exercises, including the emphasis on natural or abdominal breathing, the focused practice of reversed breathing, the gathering of *qi* in the lower cinnabar field, and some basic forms of embryo respiration (Cohen, *Way of Qigong*, 121-29). It also includes various meditations, among which "standing like a tree" is highly recommended.

Practitioners stand in one spot with their feet hip-width apart and their palms loosely facing the abdomen. They remain unmoving for ten to twenty minutes while envisioning themselves being rooted in earth and growing toward heaven, stable and strong yet swaying slightly as the *qi* passes through them. This simple standing meditation has proved effective in attention deficit and hyperactivity problems. It is also helpful in pinpointing alignment problems and strengthening the leg muscles. Other meditations are undertaken both in seated and prone positions. They may involve guiding the *qi* to specific areas of affliction or circulating it around the body in the microcosmic orbit.

The vast majority of Qigong practice consists of simple gymnastic moves that are often combined in sequences and matched with cosmological entities, such as heaven and earth, the five phases, and the eight trigrams (Jahnke, *Healing Promise*, 128). For example, a form that involves absorbing the *qi* of heaven and earth in the four directions is Wuji or Primordial Qigong, named after the Non-Ultimate at the beginning of creation. Practitioners stand facing east and breathe deeply, then raise and lower their arms and rotate their hands as they encourage the *qi* to join their bodies. They complete twelve movements of earth, repeat these in all four directions, then perform ten movements of heaven, also in all directions. The practice is deceptively simple and has a profound effect on general well-being (see www.taichi-enlightenment.com).

A form that involves engaging the *qi* of the five phases is described below. It, too, is easy to learn, involves simple, rhythmic movements, and encourages self-healing. Another popular form is called the "Eight Pieces of Brocade" (Baduan jin). Its standing version includes overhead stretches, sideways bends, arm extensions, hip circles, neck rolls, and squats, while the seated version is more meditative and teaches people to focus inward, to swallow their saliva, to guide the *qi*, and to enhance inner

Exercise: Try practicing the following Qigong sequence. How does it feel?

Five Phases Qigong

Wuji: Weight is evenly distributed among both feet. Feet are parallel and shoulder-width apart, toes on an even level. Knees are slightly bent, elbows slightly out, backs of hands face forward. The tailbone is heavy, the top of the head is light, the vertebrae of the spine are aligned.

Water—mist rises, clouds drift, soft rain falls: Inhale, as if drawn by strings, lift wrists forward, allow arms to rise to shoulder height. Hands dangle loosely, elbows bent, arms are raised. Do not raise shoulders. Exhale. Extend fingers and mentally send *qi* outward. Inhale, pull hands in towards shoulders. Exhale and lower.

Wood—roots grow into trunk and tree branches: Inhale, cup one hand within the other, both palms facing up. Raise cupped hands in front of torso, pause at chest. Exhale, turn palms down. Inhale, turn palms out and raise overhead. Exhale, separate hands and release to shoulder level, arms stretched away. Circle down and repeat.

Fire—sparks fly side to side: Inhale, draw hands near heart, palms facing each other. Move weight into right foot, turn left hip and leg out 90 degrees, lift left foot in empty step while turning palms out and extending arms. Exhale, put left foot back, shift weight to center, lower palms while bending knees. Repeat on the other side.

Earth—spread ashes, gather harvest, give outward, return to compost: Inhale, shift weight left, turn right foot out. Exhale, stretch arms into bow pose, with right arm extended, left arm bent. Inhale, draw arm in toward the heart, palms facing. Exhale, shift weight back to center. Repeat on the other side. Then inhale, turn palms up and offer hands forward, shifting weight to balls of feet. Exhale, turn palms down and sink into *Wuji*, weight at base of foot.

Metal—mine ore, gather and center: Inhale, shift weight to the left, turn body left and raise hands overhead, while lifting the right heel. Turn to center, relax heel to ground. Exhale, sink hands. Repeat on the other side.

Come back to the beginning of the cycle with **water**. End by standing in *Wuji*, observing the *qi* in the body.

centering with gentle arm circles and forward bends (Yang, *Eight Pieces*). More complex forms of Qigong include the classical Six Breaths and Five Animals' Frolic together with various new sequences: the Soaring Crane, Turtle and Snake, and Swimming Dragon (Cohen, *Way of Qigong*, ch. 12).

Beyond this, Qigong also activates a person's ability to transmit *qi* by increasing one's own store within and enhancing the sensitivity to its flow. Practitioners infuse *qi* into the body of a patient or partner, not unlike therapeutic touch in the West, to effect relaxation or healing. Used in this manner, Qigong includes forms of massage and group practice as well as the ability to send *qi* over a distance and modify *qi*-patterns by mere conscious intention (Jahnke, *Healing Promise*, ch. 14).

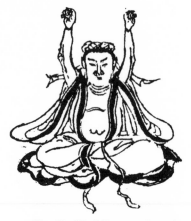

Fig. 32. "Red Dragon Stirs the Ocean": The Third Brocade.

Unlike in China, where Qigong has been praised as a miracle cure for all sorts of diseases, in the West proponents are more conservative in their claims, substantiating them with controlled studies if possible (see www. acupuncture.com/QiKung;www.tcm. edu). Conditions best studied include tension headaches, migraines, high blood pressure, respiratory conditions, post-traumatic stress syndrome, and motor problems, such as Parkinson's disease and multiple sclerosis. In general, people who join a Qigong group and practice regularly find themselves relaxed and grounded, gaining tranquility, flexibility, self-awareness, and confidence. Taught in an undemanding setting, Qigong helps in alleviating pain, increasing balance and mobility in the elderly, and giving respite to cancer patients. The exercises are gentle and easy to learn, and instructors encourage students to do what they can with ease and good cheer. They allow people to express themselves freely and find new levels of being. Often severe cases are rehabilitated with the help of patient, gentle practice (see also www.qigonginstitute.org; www.bodymindhealing.com).

One participant, for example, when asked to open her arms wide during the tree meditation realized that she had great hesitations because she could not take up that much space. This provided a completely new insight into her way of being in the world. An elderly practitioner greatly benefited from the conscious visualizations used in the Five Animals' Frolic. Plagued by arthritis in hip and knees, she would visualize herself as the ambling bear when going up stairs and as the dainty deer when descending, thus allowing her body to move more flexibly and with less pain (*Zeitschrift für Qigong Yangsheng* 2000, 2001).

Another case in point is the treatment of asthma and allergies. Here Qigong therapy involves herbal prescriptions and gentle movements together with guided breathing techniques and specific visualizations, such as the White Tiger. In the latter, patients are guided to visualize themselves in a secure, warm, protected environment, then see two white tigers approaching. The tigers represent power and protective force. Friendly and helpful, they circle the patient to establish a shield against outside demands, stresses, and allergens. Established firmly in the patient's mind, they can be called upon whenever the need arises (Cibik, *Air Passages*, 188-90).

Qigong as health practice is done by the patient for the patient. It involves effort and requires steady discipline, demanding that one take full responsibility for one's well-being. In this respect it is different from both traditional Chinese and Western medical methods and creates a new kind of patient—educated, informed, self-aware, critical, and very selective. Joining other alternative ways, its impact in the West is on the rise. An increasing number of people when faced with threatening diagnoses no longer do what the first doctor tells them, but get a second opinion. Many do not rest even then but look up their condition on the Internet and experiment with alternative methods. Qigong empowers patients and awakens them to the healing potential buried deep inside themselves. It heals and prevents diseases, a power that some envision as leading to a revolution in Western health care, overburdened by conditions that are to 70 percent preventable. Rather than living unconsciously and becoming subject to invasive medical procedures, the ideal patient of the new century keeps herself vibrantly alive through Qigong (Jahnke, *Healer Within*, 7-10; see www.feeltheqi.com).

Exercise: Go to the web (www.nqa.org; www.healerwithin.com) and find out about the organization and acceptance level of Qigong. How does it relate to mainstream medicine? What are some of the stories people tell?

Unlike the rather steady development in the West, in China Qigong has had various ups and downs, matching the political climate of the country. In the 1950s, it grew vibrantly as the state faced the dilemma of condemning Western medical methods as too bourgeois while having to provide medical services to a huge population with little resources. The government went back to traditional methods, and Qigong became part of an effort to prove that China could handle all problems on her own. In 1953, the first Qigong clinic opened in Tangshan, Hebei, followed in 1955 by one in Beidaihe near Beijing. In 1958, the Great Leap Forward encouraged peasants to forge their own steel and become industrially independent. The same local independence was also supported in health matters and about seventy new Qigong clinics opened. Following this, national Qigong conferences and officially supported training centers arose, and many new publications appeared (Despeux, "Qigong").

During the Cultural Revolution (1966-76), the Communist Party banned Qigong as feudalistic and prohibited all public practice. In 1977, when traditional practices became acceptable again, the Beijing actress Guo Lin cured herself of metastatic breast cancer with Qigong and started to teach the methods in public. In 1978, a physicist at the Shanghai Nuclear Research Institute found a material, scientific basis for *qi* in an experiment. *Qi* was defined as an electromagnetic force that could be measured and produced by a machine.

These developments opened the way for the Qigong boom of the 1980s. People were not only cured but also began to exhibit spontaneous trances, supernatural powers, and paranormal faculties. These, too, were explained scientifically and heralded as part of a new scientific revolution, which would put China at the forefront of human evolution and the pinnacle of world powers. Conferences were held, debates were opened, the Communist Party lent its support, and many leading scientists began to work on Qigong.

The Hong Kong movie industry started to produce martial arts films using Qigong methods, creating a strong pop culture and linking Qigong to exceptional abilities and feats. It was only through the movie media that martial arts came to be seen as an aspect of Qigong. At the same time, the more medical, health-oriented practices were expanded from mere breathing and gymnastics to include physical training, illness prevention, therapy, intelligence development, and supernatural faculties — i.e., penetrating vision, distant sensation, prolonged immobility, miraculously flight, walking through walls, soaring spiritually, controlling the weather, and knowing past and future.

In 1987, Yan Xin emerged. He was a Qigong master who had practiced since childhood and had learned from more than thirty masters. In a scientific experiment, he proved his ability to use external *qi* to alter the structure of water 1,500 miles away. Based on this feat, he became famous and started a lecture circuit, the so-called force-filled lectures, which were often ten hours long and attracted as many as 20,000 people. Many in the audience experienced trance reactions, spiritual experiences, spontaneous healings, and the emergence of supernatural powers. This kind of Qigong became a major craze, and Yan Xin had not only numerous followers but also people who imitated him. By 1988, over one hundred million Chinese practiced Qigong every day. Qigong masters were idolized, and the practice was taught in primary schools, professional academies, and as part of sports training.

A change occurred in the 1990s. It began gradually with the intensification of religious values in the practice and the increase in quackery, psychotic episodes, and sectarian divisions. Insufficiently trained people would teach some kind of movement and breathing to make lots of money; serious practitioners, especially of the Soaring Crane exercise, would fall into trances and not come out again, stuck in a never-never world of spontaneous movements. Masters who saw their followers and fortunes dwindle became autocratic, demanding total obedience from their followers. As a result, the political and scientific support started to wane, and there was a growing anti-Qigong polemic.

Then, in 1992, Falun dafa (Great Methods of the Dharma Wheel) arose, also known as Falun gong (www.falundafa.org). Founded by Li Hongzhi as one of thousands of Qigong groups, it soon grew to a larger entity and claimed that it was not merely a form of Qigong but represented the universal law or Buddhist dharma. Its main document *Transmitting the Dharma Wheel* (*Zhuan Falun*) appeared in 1995 on the basis of Li's lectures. It emphasizes the recovery of health, the attainment of supernatural powers, and the realization of one's spiritual nature in cosmic enlightenment. But it also includes a millenarian vision, not only presenting its practice as a major stepping stone in human evolution but actively condemning the decadence of the present age. In these aspects Falun gong is significantly different from other forms of Qigong; it broke off from the Chinese Qigong Association in 1996.

Essentially, the group's teaching centers on the idea that everyone has a "dharma wheel" (*falun*) in one's lower abdomen, just about where Daoists and Qigong followers place the cinnabar field. By nature, this wheel is dormant and has to be activated or "installed" by an enlightened master. Once it begins to rotate, it will bring about complete recovery from illness, supernatural powers, and the attainment of cosmic enlightenment. To have the dharma wheel activated, practitioners have to have the right karma that brings them in contact with Master Li. He claims to be the embodied reincarnation of a major Buddhist deity and the only living agent able to put the dharma wheel into motion. The installation of the wheel is central to the process of Falun dafa. It can be done either through a representative, a book, or a video, but ideally through Li in person. As he says in a lecture:

> We believe in predestined relationship. I can do such a thing for everyone sitting here. Right now we have only more than two thousand people. I can also do it for several thousand or more people, even over ten thousand people. That is to say, you do not need to practice at a low level. Upon purifying your bodies, and moving you up, I will install a complete cultivation practice system in your body. Right away you will practice cultivation at high levels. It will be done, however, only for practitioners who come to genuinely practice cultivation; your simply sitting here does not mean that your are a practitioner.

> Here we talk about holistically adjusting practitioners' bodies to enable you to practice cultivation. With an ill body you cannot develop cultivation energy at all. Therefore, you should not come to me for curing illnesses, and neither will I do such a thing. The primary purpose of my coming to the public is to guide people to high levels. (Li, *Zhuan Falun*, 7–8)

Falun dafa claims that once the dharma wheel begins to spin in the person's abdomen, he or she is on an accelerated track toward cosmic evolution, which leads to high moral sensitivities and great physical health. Followers of the group, to ensure this cosmic evolution, have to undertake two kinds of practices—five sets of exercises and three moral virtues. The exercises involve a set of arm stretches, a standing meditation, an up-and-down movement of the arms, a guiding of *qi* through the body by passing one's hands over it, and a sitting meditation performed in the full lotus posture. Every so often, hands are circulated over the lower abdomen, symbolizing the movement of the dharma wheel. If done properly, the exercise sequence takes about two hours.

Even more important, however, are the three moral virtues *zhen, shan, ren*—truth, goodness, forbearance—which entail being honest in all dealings, exerting kindness toward all beings, and not retaliating against wrongs. Working on these virtues, the teaching claims, will make practitioners better people, and only if they become better people can the five exercises open up their inner powers and lead them to ultimate realization.

This moral dimension of Falun dafa distinguishes it from other forms of Qigong, which tend to focus more on healing and empowerment. It may also be one of the reasons why Falun dafa was so successful, given the ethical vacuum of post-communist China.

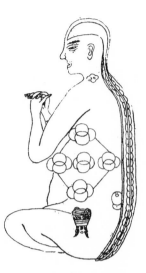

Fig. 33. Daoist alchemical reactions in the area of the dharma wheel.

Followers of the movement, although organized in small groups that function independently, are closely tied to the teaching because any practice other than Falun dafa is believed to stop the dharma wheel from turning, and Li Hongzhi will not activate it a second time. Also, as the dedicated practice of the exercises is supposed to heal all ailments, followers are discouraged from using medical advice and professional services. Their intense gratitude toward Li Hongzhi (who now lives in the U.S.) as well as their personal healing experiences and improvements have led to a strong veneration of the leader as a living buddha.

This veneration, together with followers' refusal to participate in certain aspects of society have caused the Chinese government to perceive Falun gong as a cult that threatens inner security and political stability. As a result, since the summer of 1999, when several tens of thousands of followers protested against discrimination, Falun dafa has been outlawed and its followers persecuted, often violently and with torture.

Exercise: Discuss the "cult" nature of Falun dafa. Go to the web (www. religioustolerance.org) and find out what makes a religious movement a cult. If found a cult, should it be radically suppressed? Or is the government overreacting?

The government's condemnation and persecution of Falun dafa has had a serious impact on Chinese cultivation practices. All forms of Qigong and even some schools of Taiji quan have become suspect in China, making healing practices once again the victim of politics and creating an atmosphere of distrust and fear among practitioners. Many Qigong clinics are closed and even though practices continue both in public and in private, Qigong and Taiji quan are not as popular as they once were. On the other hand, they survive and flourish greatly outside of China and are becoming increasingly a main staple of Western practices.

Further Readings

Chang, Stephen T. 1986. *The Complete System of Self-Healing: Internal Exercise*. San Francisco: Tao Publishing.

Cibik, Ted J. 2003. *Air Passages: Surviving Asthma Naturally*. Leechburg, Penn.: Oak Tree Productions.

Cohen, Kenneth S. 1997. *The Way of Qigong: The Art and Science of Chinese Energy Healing*. New York: Ballantine.

Despeux, Catherine. 2003. "Qigong—Ein Ausdruck des modernen China." *Zeitschrift für Qigong Yangsheng* 2003, 57-66.

Jahnke, Roger. 1997. *The Healer Within: Using Traditional Chinese Techniques to Release Your Body's Own Medicine*. San Francisco: HarperCollins.

_____. 2002. *The Healing Promise of Qi: Creating Extraordinary Wellness Through Qigong and Tai Chi*. New York: Contemporary Books.

MacRitchie, James. 1997. *The Chi Kung Way*. San Francisco: HarperCollins.

Miura, Kunio. 1989. "The Revival of Qi: Qigong in Contemporary China." In *Taoist Meditation and Longevity Techniques*, edited by L. Kohn, 329-58. Ann Arbor: University of Michigan, Center for Chinese Studies Publications.

Xin, Yan. 1997. *Secrets and Benefits of Internal Qigong Cultivation*. Malvern, Penn.: Amber Leaf Press.

Yang, Jwing-ming. 1988. *The Eight Pieces of Brocade: Improving and Maintaining Health*. Jamaica Plain, Mass.: Yang's Martial Arts Association.

Chapter 18
Taiji Quan and Martial Arts

Taiji quan, also spelled T'ai Chi Ch'uan, means "Great Ultimate Boxing." It goes back to the seventeenth century when it arose from a combination of philosophy, gymnastics, and martial training. An integrated flow of moves, stretches, squats, and kicks, Taiji quan is oriented geographically and begins and ends either facing east or south. Its forms can be as long as 108 moves, which have rather fanciful names, such as "grasp the bird's tail," "single whip," "playing the lute," "high pet the horse," and "embrace tiger, return to mountain." Often quite complex, the forms take regular, long-term practice to master. They are executed while standing: knees bent, the stomach pulled in, back straight, head up, and hands and feet moving from the abdomen rather than from the shoulders and hips. The eyes see straight ahead without looking at anything in particular. The mind is empty but attentive, relaxed but alert, open to outside stimuli but without reaction. From a calm mind focused intention arises which in turn leads to harmonious *qi*-flow.

It is best to practice at times of rising *qi*, i.e., in the early morning hours. Practitioners dress in loose clothing and wear flexible shoes. Some forms also add an instrument, such as a sword, a staff, a pole, or a spear. Usually done outdoors and in a natural setting, Taiji quan is not accompanied by music or other extraneous supports. Rather, it invites the cosmic harmony of nature into the body-mind. The breath is through the nose: deep and abdominal. As it is physiologically impossible to be stressed and breathe deeply at the same time, Taiji quan has a calming effect, opens the body and stills the mind. Long-term practice leads to a sense of inner spontaneity, a continuous flowing movement of self and universe, a freedom from judgment and urgency, and an appearance of softness and innocence (Delza, *T'ai Chi Ch'uan Experience*). As Agnes Lee says:

> When one is actually practicing the exercise, ego anxieties about the past and the future are eliminated by the attention necessary in order to stay in the immediacy of first this movement and then that movement and then always again this

movement and then that movement. ("Movement Within Still-ness," 30)

While the bulk of Taiji quan is individual in orientation, there is also a form of partner practice known as "push-hands" (*tuishou*). Done with one other person, this is usually limited to four basic moves — ward-off, roll-back, press, and push. Two practitioners face each other, coordinate their breathing, and in a steady rhythm, which can be slower or faster,

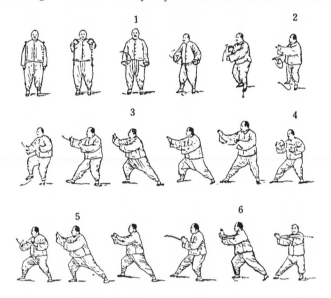

Fig. 34. A Taiji quan sequence.

push against each other using Taiji moves. It is best to practice push-hands with many different partners to develop sensitivity and the ability to respond to any force. Push-hands not only increases the depth of one's personal practice but can also be applied fruitfully in one's daily life.

One may well be pushed on the street, on the bus, on the job, or in the family, and the primary inclination is always to push back. Through the practice, adepts realize that the most effective way to neutralize a push is to open and lean back and allow the incoming *qi* to dissipate. As a result, instead of expanding a great deal of energy throwing themselves at bar-riers and engaging in conflicts, practitioners develop an inner peaceful-ness and stability, a collected calmness that will allow them to deal with situations profitably and efficiently (Jou, *Dao of Taijiquan*).

In addition to its self-defense and meditational qualities, Taiji quan also has a healing effect. Several controlled studies have shown marked improvement in patients with Parkinson's diseases as well as in seniors struggling with imbalance, dizziness, and vertigo. Regular practice increases the circulation, harmonizes the respiration, strengthens the muscles, enhances muscle control, straightens the spine, opens the chest, and increases balance. It can also alleviate chronic conditions, such as high blood pressure, anemia, joint problems, indigestion, asthma, sciatica, tuberculosis, heart ailments, eye and skin diseases, as well as mental and emotional disturbances. It is also, though not sweaty and exhausting, a fat burner—using up as many calories as downhill skiing. Psychologically Taiji quan with its calm and graceful moves reduces stress and nervous dispositions, while increasing harmony, providing a sense of wholeness, and creating a feeling of inner quiet and equanimity. Practitioners feel refreshed and energized after their daily routine, the body pulsating with warm and strong *qi*. They can face the world with confidence and ease, and as a result live happier and longer lives.

Exercise: Go to the web (www.taoist.org.english; www.worldtaijiday.org; www.taiji. org) and look for studies on the medical effects of Taiji quan. What conditions has Taiji quan been linked with? Where is it most efficient? Are there controlled studies on its effects? Any theories on how it heals?

Historically, Taiji quan has its roots among healing gymnastics, Daoist philosophy, and martial training. Its gymnastic roots are obvious in the emphasis on deep, abdominal breathing; the gentleness of the moves; the rhythmic alternation of bends and stretches; and the fanciful names of its moves that are often associated with animals. Many of its patterns are similar to Qigong exercises and integrate the *daoyin* models of old, causing Taiji quan to harmonize *qi*-flow, enhance blood circulation, release stress, and improve balance and health.

The philosophical roots of Taiji quan are found in the concept of the Great Ultimate (*taiji*), a name for the universe at the time of creation, when yin and yang are present but are not yet differentiated into the five phases. Daoist and Neo-Confucian thinkers of the Song dynasty (960-1260) describe the Great Ultimate as arising from the Non-Ultimate (*wuji*), commonly depicted as an empty circle. This represents the world before creation, at its most primordial. After evolving, the Great Ultimate, shown as interlocking patterns of black and white or yin and yang, it develops the universe through the interaction of the five phases. From this basis, religious practitioners strive for a reunification with the state of creation, hoping to revert the process of evolution.

This recovery of primordial union is visually depicted in the *Diagram of the Great Ultimate Explained* (*Taiji tushuo*) by Zhou Dunyi (1017–1073). It shows several empty circles underneath the five phases. For practice, this means that adepts identify the flow of the five phases in their bodies, then sublimate them into yin and yang and from there unify all into a flow of pure primordial *qi*. The philosophy of the Great Ultimate provides the rationale for Taiji quan as a moving meditation, whose ultimate goal is a return to the origins, accompanied by the creation of inner, cosmic harmony (www.eng.taoism.org.hk).

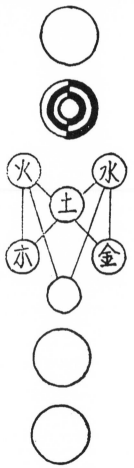

The popular symbol of the Great Ultimate, the well-known yin-yang diagram consisting of a circle with black and white curved halves is a later expression of this philosophy. Grown from ancient arrangements of the trigrams of the *Book of Changes*, it goes back to the sixteenth century, when more static depictions of the Great Ultimate and other cosmological ideas were merged with artistic depictions of cosmic energy, usually shown in rings of clouds and whirling spirals. The Taiji diagram was published in 1613, greatly influencing the intellectual world at the time (Louis, "The Genesis of an Icon"). It is no accident, therefore, that the early martial creators of Taiji quan in the seventeenth century picked up on the Great Ultimate and its popular symbol to signify the cosmic dimension of their art.

Fig. 35. The Diagram of the Great Ultimate.

In its martial roots, Taiji quan goes back to the need for self-defense among Chinese communities and temples. The most famous warrior monks were those of the Buddhist Shaolin Temple (near Luoyang), associated with the legendary Bodhidharma, the sixth-century founder of

Chinese Chan Buddhism (www.aboutshaolin.com). Monks of the temple — as well as Daoists and peasants — helped the Tang rulers to win the empire in the early seventh century. However, after this records do not show any military activity at Shaolin. On the contrary, in the thirteenth century, the monastery was easily sacked by Mongol troops. This changed in the sixteenth century, when the Ming dynasty was in decline and looting bandits and marauding armies made self-defense a priority. The Shaolin monks became famous for their fighting skills, especially with the staff. Unarmed combat (*quan*, lit. "fist") became dominant only in the seventeenth century, when the incoming Qing dynasty prohibited all use of weapons among non-military fighters. Both monastic and civil militias accordingly developed new techniques, combining defensive moves with the age-old practices of longevity breathing and gymnastics (Shahar, "Ming-Period Evidence").

The newly emerging techniques were then linked with the most famous patriarchs of the monastic schools — with the Buddhist patriarch Bodhidharma, who was duly credited with the *Sinews Transformation Classic* (*Yijin jing*), and the Daoist immortal Zhang Sanfeng, a largely legendary figure whose life, works, and methods became known through trance-induced channeling (Wong, *Investigations*). While there were many practices of this sort, Taiji quan as we know it was created by the military officer Chen Wangting. When the Qing conquest was complete in 1644, he retired to his hometown and began to teach martial gymnastics consisting of five routines and a sequence of 108 moves. His methods were transmitted through the family and organized into a slightly less martial system by his descendant Chen Zhangxing (1771-1853). The practice, known today as the Chen style, emphasizes relaxation and softness and consists of a series of rather simple moves in the four directions. Keeping the practitioner moving at all times, the practice demands concentration and alertness, insisting on inner as well as physical competence.

A second major form of Taiji quan is the Yang style, a derivative from the Chen style. It was created by Yang Luchan (1799-1872), who originally studied Shaolin boxing then visited the Chen family and became a student of Chen Zhangxing. Small in stature but strong in practice, he soon rose to be head disciple. Stories tell of his prowess and agility, how he could gracefully lift articles by only lightly touching them with his spear, and how he could stop a fire by tearing down a wall with a mere touch. He also could shoot arrows with his plain fingers, always hitting the target. He was so agile that when his daughter once slipped with a basin of water in her hands, he not only caught her but also the basin, and not a drop of water was spilled (Wile, *T'ai Chi Touchstones*).

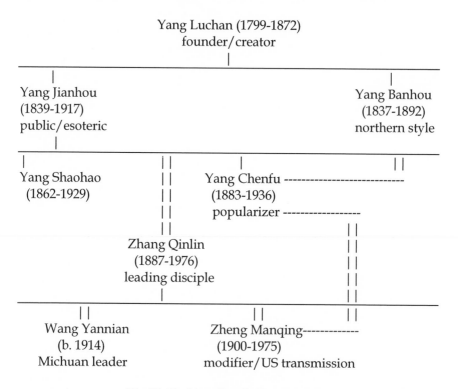

Fig. 36. The Yang Family Taiji Lineage.

Yang Luchan had three sons. The oldest died in infancy, but the other two grew up to become leading Taiji quan masters. Yang Banhou (1837-1892) started out being rather martial, then gradually learned to appreciate the more meditative quality of the practice. Yang Jianhou (1839-1917) became his father's true heir. He was an expert in empty-handed forms as well as in sword and spear practice, and trained numerous students. His son Yang Chenfu (1883-1936) was his main disciple together with Zhang Qinlin (1887-1976), who came to the Yang family as gardener at the age of twelve. He practiced throughout his life and was known for his prowess and agility. Their main students were Zheng Manqing (1900-1975) and Wang Yannian (b. 1914) who made Yang-style practice the predominant form of Taiji quan today, both in China and the U.S. They each condensed and modified it further, making the practice soft and rounded, with wide arm movements, circular patterns, and intricate flexings in the wrists and arms. Both had various students, among whom T. T. Liang (1897-1999) is best known in the West (see Liang, *T'ai Chi Ch'uan*). Wang Yannian, moreover, has taught an esoteric (*michuan*) version of the Yang style, both unarmed and with swords and staffs (Rodell, *Chinese Swordsmanship*).

The third major form of Taiji quan is the Wu style, founded by Wu Yuxiang (1812-1880), a student of both Chen Zhangxing and Yang Luchan. He developed a more martial version of the practice, which includes kicks and fierce, pointed moves. Typically Wu-style Taiji quan uses four parts to every move and pose: start, connect, open, and close. Starting is undertaken while standing still; it serves to create the intended move mentally in one's intention. Connecting, the phase from Wuji to Taiji, gets the body ready to move in the desired direction. Opening is the initial attack, hold, or retreat. Closing, finally, is the part when the move is fully executed and the practitioner returns again to stillness.

Through its martial roots, Taiji quan not only furthered strength, discipline, and willpower but also inherited the two main lineages of Chinese martial thinking. They are ancient Confucian chivalry, which encouraged the practice of archery and charioteering as tools for aristocratic self-cultivation and which emphasized honor, respect, good manners, precise timing, balance, and composure in all actions; and the tradition of bending and softness of ancient Daoism, expressed most clearly in Sunzi's *Art of War*, which stressed flexibility, yielding, humility, nonviolence, inner focus, and wisdom (Rodell, *Chinese Swordsmanship*, 3-6). Taiji quan arose through the combination of these traits with the practice of healing gymnastics and the philosophy of the Great Ultimate. It thereby evolved from mere martial training to a leading martial art, i.e., using the qualities of combat training for spiritual pursuits (Raposa, *Meditation and the Martial Arts*).

Martial arts emphasize character building as much as physical development, insisting on a strong moral base and nonviolent outlook, deep respect for others and unfailing obedience, discipline and honorable conduct, inner stillness and single-minded dedication, humility and acceptance, as well as a letting go of ego and the unfolding of inner calmness and stability which lead to utter fearlessness and a sense of being centered in the universe (see Kauz, Becker in Nelson, *Martial Arts Reader*, 79-95, 97-110). They guide people toward health and wholeness, physical vigor and well-being, joined by a deep respect for life and a sense of cosmic unity.

Martial arts are spiritual as well as health practices, and as such differ significantly from competitive sports and/or military training. Practitioners have the knowledge and ability to seriously injure or even kill an opponent, notably through the practice of *dimmak*, the "death touch" or momentary blockage of vital meridian points at a critical time in *qi*-flow (Walker and Bauer, *Ancient Art*). Still, they strictly emphasize nonviolence, and many stories tell of incidents where a martial arts practitioner who easily could have flattened the aggressor defused a potentially violent situation with calmness, patience, and kindness (see Dobson, Funakoshi in Nelson, *Martial Arts Handbook*, 113-16, 117-22).

> **Exercise:** Reflect on the understanding of martial and military in the West. What are the first associations that come to mind? How are they seen in our culture? What virtues and negative traits do we see in martial training?

Once established, Taiji quan developed an extensive body of literature. Texts on the practice can be divided into four groups. First, there are the ancient Taiji classics, which include the *Taiji quan Classic* (*Taiji quan jing*), the *Taiji quan Treatise* (*Taiji quan lun*), the *Mental Elucidation of the Thirteen Postures* (*Shisan shixing zhi xinming*), and the *Song of the Thirteen Postures* (*Shisan shixing ge*) (see Liang, *T'ai Chi Ch'uan*; Lo and Inn, *Essence*; Davis, *Taijiquan Classics*).

Ascribed to legendary figures like Zhang Sanfeng or by anonymous authors, these texts go back to the seventeenth and eighteenth centuries. They tend to be short verses that focus on general principles and the definition of major terms, such as bending, yielding, and balance. They refer to the Non-Ultimate and to yin and yang, but are predominantly practical in outlook. They also emphasize the concept of *jin*, literally "sinews," which in Taiji literature indicates the physical and mental force, the intention and *qi* as evident in one's movements. It is very important to *fajin*, "bring forth sinews energy," since it shows that one's practice is rooted in the depth of one's being and is not merely a formal repetition of outward moves.

A second group of Taiji quan texts are the transmissions of the Yang family, from the nineteenth and early twentieth century (Wile, *T'ai-Chi Touchstones*). Including short written treatises and oral transmissions of Yang Banhou and his son Chenfu, they consist of more extensive practical instructions, advice on how to deal with opponents, and stories about the practice of the masters. From the same period is a third group of texts, which include materials from both the Yang and other Taiji schools, which Douglas Wile has translated in his *Lost T'ai-Chi Classics*. The texts here are longer and more detailed, and their tendency is to refer more to philosophical concepts and issues, involving theories from ancient Daoism and the *Book of Changes*. There is a distinct unfolding in the worldview of Taiji quan toward a wider, more encompassing perspective and deeper philosophical speculation.

The fourth and last group of Taiji writings are of the twentieth century and include the works of Cheng Manqing, T. T. Liang, Jou Tsung-Hwa, and Wang Yannian. It is interesting to note that all left mainland China after the Communist take-over in 1949, and that Cheng, Liang, and Jou came to the practice of Taiji quan because of illness.

Cheng had a accident as a child which left him slightly disabled, then contracted tuberculosis in his twenties. Only after he began to practice Taiji quan with diligence did his condition improve. He was a teacher of traditional Chinese arts, calligraphy, and poetry, worked as a doctor of Chinese medicine for a time, and had a great interest in Western science. His writings reflect his erudition. Besides detailed, illustrated practice instructions and subtle commentaries on the ancient Taiji classics, they include treatises on the medical efficacy of Taiji quan and its power to connect people to the source, as well as on the physics of strength and balance and the psychology of fear (Lo and Inn, *Ch'eng Tzu*, 75-81; Wile, *Cheng Man Ch'ing's Instructions*).

T. T. Liang, too, began his practice after a grave illness, then moved on to become a full-time teacher of Taiji quan. He moved from Taiwan to New England in the early 1960s, where he taught numerous students until his death at the age of 102. His writings include practice instructions, explanations of terms and techniques, comments on mental and meditational practice, as well as personal notes and remembrances. He also developed a particular Taiji quan philosophy of his own, formulating a set of guiding principles that helped him both in self-cultivation and social interaction.

Exercise: Reflect on the role of disease in the unfolding of spirituality and self-cultivation. Do you know of any cases where people came to religion because of illness in other religions and countries? What does your culture say about the relationship of sickness/suffering and otherworldly attainments?

Jou Tsung-Hwa began the practice of Taiji quan in 1964 at age 47, when he was diagnosed with an incurable heart condition. He studied the styles of all three schools and developed his own methods. Coming to the U.S. in 1971 to obtain a doctorate in mathematics, he began to attract students and remained an active teacher until his death in 1998. He also initiated the Zhang Sanfeng Festival, a large gathering of Taiji quan practitioners which is held every year in June in northern Pennsylvania (www.americansocietyofinternalarts.com). His work includes practice instructions together with notes on the history, philosophy, and cosmology of the practice (Jou, *Dao of Taijiquan*).

Wang Yannian is best known for his transmission of the *michuan* (esoteric) Yang style. Born in 1914, he came to Taiji quan on the basis of military training. He graduated from police academy in 1932, then fought as a colonel in the Sino-Japanese war (1937-1945) and the civil war between nationalists and communists (1945-1949). After fleeing to Taiwan, he served in the self-defense force and began to teach Taiji quan. He still continues to work out with people in the park on a daily basis and has inspired various Taiji quan organizations, both in Taiwan and overseas.

In the U.S., Wang is the central focus of the American Yangjia Michuan Taijiquan Association (www.aymta.org). Their magazine, *AYMTA Journal*, since 1993 has recorded trends in the form and methods of teaching. Its 2000 issue (vol. 8, no.2) is dedicated to the fiftieth anniversary of Wang's teaching career and contains a documentation of his life as well as an interview, an account of the life of his teacher Zhang Qinlin (who died, sick and impoverished, in 1976 at the end of the Cultural Revolution), as well as several accounts of students' experiences with the master.

The journal also provides advice and insights on teaching. For example, a recent issue asks about possible blockages in people's progress. Teachers, mostly from Europe, respond by referring to mental obstacles, such as pride, self-importance, and rigidity. "Too many emotions, too much thinking during the practice," Sabine Metzle says, "leads to the separation of body and mind instead of unifying them. Too much will to progress, to obtain results instead of letting go" is a great hindrance. It can be eased by cultivating calm self-awareness and being in the present (vol. 10, no.2: 28). All physical difficulties, however awkward, should be taken with patience and remedied with an enduring trust in the spiritual unfolding of the practice, which as Bede Bidlack notes, eventually leads to a state of self-forgetfulness and spontaneous oneness with the flow of the Dao (vol. 11, no.1: 17). The gentle, flowing practice eventually encourages the body to move in perfect coordination, creating a powerful harmony in body and mind. Sophia Delza describes it in a poem:

> Creating calm, longevity,
> Keener insight and awareness
> To society and self, T'ai Chi Ch'uan
> Completes a circle, expressed
> In form and motion—
> With time not counting time,
> Returning to the point where it began,
> With consciousness enlivened,
> Finding, in the end, a new beginning.
> (*T'ai Chi Ch'uan Experience*, 223)

Further Readings

Cheng, Man-Ching. 1985. *Cheng Tzu's Thirteen Treatises on T'ai Chi Chuan*. Berkeley: North Atlantic Books.

Davis, Barbara. 2004. *The Taiji quan Classics: An Annotated Translation*. Berkeley: North Atlantic Books.

Delza, Sophia. 1996. *The T'ai-Chi Ch'uan Experience*. Albany: State University of New York Press.

Lee, Agnes C.J. 1987. "Movement With Stillness and Stillness Within Man: The Contemplative Character of T'ai Chi Chuan." *Ching Feng* 30: 25-38.

Liang, T. T. 1977. *T'ai Chi Ch'uan for Health and Self-Defense*. New York: Vintage Books.

Lo, Benjamin, and Martin Inn. 1979. *The Essence of T'ai Chi Ch'uan*. Berkeley: North Atlantic Books.

_____. 1985. *Cheng Tzu's Thirteen Classics on T'ai Chi Ch'uan*. Berkeley: North Atlantic Books.

Louis, Francois. 2003. "The Genesis of an Icon: The Taiji Diagram's Early History." *Harvard Journal of Asiatic Studies* 63: 145-96.

Nelson, Randy F., ed. 1989. *Martial Arts Reader*. Woodstock, NY: Overlook Press.

Raposa, Michael L. 2003. *Meditation and the Martial Arts*. Charleston: University of Virginia Press.

Rodell, Scott M. 2003. *Chinese Swordsmanship: The Yang Family Taiji Jian Tradition*. Annandale, Virg.: Seven Stars Trading Co.

Shahar, Meir. 2001. "Ming-Period Evidence of Shaolin Martial Practice." *Harvard Journal of Asiatic Studies* 61: 359-413.

Walker, A. Flane, and Richard C. Bauer. 2002. *The Ancient Art of Life and Death: The Book of Dim Mak*. Boulder: Paladin Press.

Wile, Douglas. 1983. *T'ai-Chi Touchstones: Yang Family Secret Transmission*. New York: Sweet Chi Press.

_____. 1985. *Cheng Man-Ching's Advanced Tai-Chi Form Instructions*. New York: Sweet Chi Press.

_____. 1996. *Lost Tai-Chi Classics from the Late Ching Dynasty*. Albany: State University of New York Press.

Wong, Shiu Hon. 1982. *Investigations into the Authenticity of the Chang San-feng ch'uan-chi*. Canberra: Australian National University Press.

Chapter 19

Meditation

Meditation is a state of mind where ego-related concerns and critical evaluations are suspended in favor of perceiving a deeper, subtler, and possibly divine flow of consciousness. The body is held very still and thoughts are calmed or ignored. The mind is quiet and attention is focused on one object. This object can be a single, moving or unmoving entity, a general openness to all sensory stimuli, or a specific scene or sequence of events.

When the object is a single entity, we speak of concentrative meditation. Its practice involves one-pointedness of mind, complete control of attention, and the absorption in a single object to the exclusion of all else. The object can be a sound or mantra, a visual diagram, or a concrete object (e.g., flame, vase, deity). Beginners in most traditions start with the breath, observing it with the help of counting either the number or the length of respirations. The goal here is to still the conscious mind so that the subtle murmur of the subconscious and unconscious can be perceived and the true nature of consciousness reveals itself.

> **Exercise:** Sit comfortably with back straight. Close or lower your eyes. Take a few deep breaths. Then begin by counting to four as you inhale, and again count to four as you exhale. Continue for five to ten minutes. See what this practice does to your mind and body.

When the object of meditation is a general openness to all sorts of sensory stimuli, we speak of insight meditation. This encourages a sense of free-flowing awareness, detached observation, and attentive mindfulness. Insight meditation usually begins with the recognition of physical sensations and subtle events in the body. It also involves paying attention to reactions to outside stimuli, recognizing but not evaluating them. Often associated with notions of deeper understanding or wisdom, it encourages the appreciation of life as a flow and leads practitioners to see the body as an unstable, ever-changing energetic entity.

Should the meditator focus on a specific scene or sequence of events, we speak of visualization. This form involves envisioning energy flows, deities, cosmic patterns, saints' lives, or potential future events. The scenes are either seen with complete detachment or involve the participation of the practitioner. In either case, visualization opens the consciousness to more subtle levels, allowing the powers of the unconscious to manifest themselves and bringing new dimensions to the practitioner's life.

Meditation can be both pleasurable and an excruciating effort, especially if the mind wanders and is swamped with thoughts or the body is in discomfort from prolonged sitting. It is a form self-hypnosis, with a clear outline of goals and the subtle creation of personal suggestions. Goals come in three types. In modern Western societies, meditation primarily serves for self-improvement, be it in the form of healing, stress-reduction, pain-management, increased productivity, or a general calming of the mind. For example, concentration exercises create better efficiency at work, insight meditation eliminates unwanted emotional baggage, and visualization can help in healing, pain-control, and past-life regressions, as well as sports training and business management.

A second kind of goal appears in traditional cultures and religions, where meditation—often joined by devotion—forms a major path to connect with the divine and to realize spiritual goals. The mental calmness it provides and the access it offers to the subtler levels of consciousness serve to awaken a greater power or universal force—defined by different traditions as God, Dao, âtman, or buddhanature. Meditation suspends conscious and ego-related thinking and thereby allows the divine or cosmic powers to come to the fore, expands the vision and understanding of the practitioner and eventually transforms him or her from an ordinary to a sagely or enlightened person.

A third major goal of meditation appears in destructive cults, where it is used to brainwash followers into dependence on the cult leader. Often combined with a poor diet, sleep deprivation, acts of humiliation, and a lack of privacy, meditation can become a strong tool of mind control and a key vehicle of indoctrination and personal dependence. Determined in content and methodology by the cult leader, meditation in this context leaves no personal freedom to the follower and unfortunately often succeeds in the complete abolition of his or her critical thinking and sense of self-preservation (Hassan, *Cult Mind Control*).

In all these different modes of meditation, the suspension of ego-related concerns and critical, intellectual evaluations forms a cornerstone of the practice and is the basis of its success. However, there is a distinct difference in degree. In its contemporary application as a way toward self-improvement and healing, critical evaluation is only suspended very lightly during the actual practice and remains strong otherwise. The entire practice, after all, is motivated and framed in terms of egotistic concerns and personal interests.

Traditional religions typically set harsh tests before they teach meditation and warn people off rather than encourage them. Practitioners have the clear and conscious intention to suspend their egos in order to attain a deeper, personal religious experience — defined in the terms of their creed and often involving an encompassing awareness of the divine and a consciousness of detached altruism or compassion. In cultic contexts, finally, the suspension of ego-based thinking is made permanent and replaced with a brain-washed dependency on the cult's doctrines and the leader's orders. Apparent benefits of this state include freedom from personal responsibility and decision-making, a sense of immersion in the group, a lack of doubt, and a feeling of belonging. Although it may feel good at first, this state of dependency and uncritical surrender is harmful in the long run and often leads to ill health and psychological trauma.

The vast majority of Westerners who practice meditation use it for health and self-improvement. They keep the practice free from doctrines and do not follow a guru or movement, but undertake it by themselves and in limited amounts, maybe twenty minutes once or twice a day rather than in week- and month-long retreats. Modern science recognizes this way of meditating as an important factor in healing and has found that especially concentration practice, as described in Herbert Benson's *The Relaxation Response*, is very beneficial for healing. Calm thoughts and concentrated breathing induce a relaxed state and deeper blood oxygenation. As a result, the heart rate decreases, urgencies diminish, and there is less overall tension (see also library.thinkquest.org; www.crystalclarity.com).

Meditation also has an effect on the endocrine system, reducing the concentration of stress hormones, such as lactate, cortisol, and epinephrine in the bloodstream, while increasing melatonin which enhances good cheer, maintains health, and prevents disease. In terms of brain activity, studies have clearly shown that concentration practitioners emit calm, steady alpha waves, while advanced practitioners show a predominance of theta waves, which indicate a restful, sleeplike yet conscious state. The frontal lobes of the brain are deactivated, and there is less activity in the parietal lobe. As a result, practitioners are able to immerse themselves in the present and do less judging and striving than non-meditators (Shapiro and Walsh, *Meditation*). It has also become clear that insight meditation shifts amygdala activity in the prefrontal cortex toward the left, indicative of relaxed, enthusiastic, and energized states (Goleman, *New York Times*, 4 Feb. 2003).

Visualization, finally, has proven successful in creating a positive outlook and sense of hope. This is especially useful in cancer treatments, where people's thinking often is that "cancer means death" or that it "cannot be controlled." Replacing these thoughts with positive enhancements and visions of oneself as healthy can make the difference between life and death (Simonton, *Getting Well Again*; Samuels, *Seeing With the Mind's Eye*). In all its forms, meditation calms and restores people, empowers patients, and teaches them to see themselves as participating in their health by creating their own state of mind, attitude, and bodily reality. It provides a positive way to work with all sorts of life situations and especially sickness and disease. Rather than seeing ill health as a dangerous enemy that has to be defeated, it becomes an indicator of imbalance in the body and a potential chance for getting time off, being pampered, and reviewing one's activities and needs. Releasing tension from the mind and encouraging positive attitudes, meditation is a great aide to healing.

> **Exercise:** Go to the web (www.meditationcenter.com; www.learningmeditation.com; www.meditationsociety.com) and look up some recent studies on the physiology and psychology of meditation. What types of meditation are currently being studied? What are the main trends in meditation research? What kinds of studies do you think should be undertaken?

The Daoist tradition is familiar with all three kinds of meditation, both for healing and spiritual goals. The Qigong meditation "standing like a pine tree" is a good example of concentration practice; Taiji quan with its emphasis on open awareness and letting go is a form of insight meditation in motion; and the active guidance of *qi* in gymnastics and Qigong to specific areas of the body is a basic form of visualization. However, beyond this modern application of meditation in healing, the Daoist tradition has also applied all three forms, gearing them to the creation of higher awareness and oneness with the Dao. They are still being practiced actively and represented by various organizations in the U.S. (www.abodetao.com; www.daoistcenter.org; www.daoiststudies.org).

Beginning from a base of good health that was reached through medical treatments, a change in diet, and the practice of gymnastics and breathing, Daoist meditation guides the adept toward transformation into a cosmic being, a transcendent or immortal. An immortal in Daoism is a human being who through a certain training attains youthfulness, longevity, and mystical freedom on this earth, followed by ascent into heaven and continuous paradisiacal ease and splendor.

Immortality as a process can be divided into three aspects of transformation: in terms of body, emotions, and consciousness. Perception of the body changes from an individual, personal entity to being part of a larger natural framework in oneness with the cosmos. No longer a means toward sensory gratification, the body becomes a vehicle of perfection. Similarly, a distance is established toward desires and emotions, which are found unconnected to the underlying truth of the Dao and come to be seen as mere surface waves. Worldly attainments, cravings, and pursuits are seen as shallow and even considered hindrances to the goal. Last but not least, the conscious mind changes from being occupied by "foolish imaginings" and ordinary thoughts to a means for penetrating the mystery of the all-encompassing source. Altogether, the understanding of oneself as an individual with a specific body, a set personality, and individual thought patterns is replaced by a wider sense of oneness with the Dao.

The most basic Daoist meditation is concentration, already practiced among self-cultivation adepts in ancient China (see Roth, *Original Tao*). It teaches adepts to focus their attention on the breath as it expands and contracts the diaphragm, centering their awareness in the lower cinnabar field. The goal is to attain full control over the conscious mind, gaining the ability to fixate it on whatever object they wish for any length of time and thereby realizing perfect tranquility of the will and the intention (see Kohn, *Seven Steps to the Tao*).

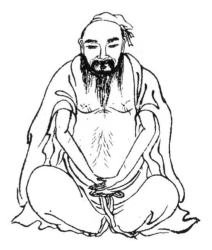

Fig. 37. A Daoist practicing concentration.

Another concentration method is "guarding the One" or "maintaining oneness" (*shouyi*). Here the adept focuses all attention on one bodily center or deity within, hoping to attain total absorption and a sense of oneness. The earliest form of guarding the One is concentration on the inner organs with the goal of keeping the *qi* in them. The result is not only long life but control over all bodily functions and appearances, which will eventually lead to the freedom of immortality (Kohn, *Taoist Meditation*).

The modern version of Daoist concentration practice is quiet sitting (*jing-zuo*). It consists of sitting or kneeling quietly, preferably in a special meditation hut or chamber, and focusing one's attention on the breath. Regulating the breath and following it deep into the abdomen to gain control over the diaphragm, the Ocean of *Qi* is activated. Once the diaphragm is fully controlled, breathing is reversed, i.e., the diaphragm rises on the inhalation, breaths become deeper and less frequent, and eventually a hot *qi* is felt to fill the abdomen. This *qi* then, without conscious help, rises up into the spine and moves around the body in the microcosmic orbit. The practice creates a deep inner state of absorption.

Insight meditation is the second level of Daoist meditation. Based on Buddhist *vipassana*, it is called "inner observation" (*neiguan*) and encourages the open appreciation of all sensory data together with the calm, intentional awareness of the different parts and activities of the body, ultimately resulting in a state of no-mind and nonaction. To enter the insight phase, adepts use the stability of mind gained in concentration to critically examine their body-mind. Already trained in the religious worldview, they come to understand that their conscious mind is originally part of universal spirit which works through the human mind and governs life perfectly, but—due to delusion—is wasted on sensory amusements and the uncontrolled exertions of eyes, ears, mouth, nose, body, and mind. This is the underlying reason for passions and desires. As the *Scripture of Inner Observation* (*Neiguan jing*) says:

> Spirit is neither black nor white, neither red nor yellow, neither big nor small, neither short nor long, neither crooked nor straight, neither soft nor hard, neither thick nor thin, neither round nor square. It goes on changing and transforming without measure, merges with yin and yang, greatly encompasses heaven and earth, subtly enters the tiniest blade of grass.

> Controlled, it is straightforward; let loose, it goes mad. Purity and tranquility make it live, defilements and nervousness cause it to perish. When shining it can illuminate the eight

ends of the universe. When darkened it will go wrong even in one single direction. You need only keep it empty and still, then life and the Dao will spontaneously be permanent. (Kohn, *Taoist Meditation*, 207)

In a similar way, the physical body is originally a microcosmic replica of the cosmos and forms part of the continuous natural transformations of *qi*, moving along naturally and perfectly if left to its own devices. However, people identify with sensory data and create an artificial identity, which then judges and evaluates, develops desires and aversions, and resists the natural flow. Any constructed identity or "personal body" comes to be, as the *Book of the Dao and the Virtue* says, "the reason why I have terrible vexations. If I did not have a personal body, what vexations would I have?" (ch. 13) The more one identifies with this personal body, the farther one removes from the Dao. The more one practices inner observation, on the other hand, the easier it is to move beyond the limited self and gain universal being. The resulting personality is unbound by physical limitations, emotional values, and conscious classifications. Any conscious ego identity that was there before is lost, and it becomes hard to determine at what point the individual ends and the Dao begins.

> **Exercise:** Examine yourself and distinguish the personal body and the physical body in your experience. For example, is the need for sweets a learned, personal trait or an instinctive, natural aspect? Is it possible to reduce ourselves back from the personal body to a more simple, physical level? What would that involve?

The highest level of Daoist meditation is visualization. Used to focus *qi* in the body and enhance the vitality of the organs, its full expression involves visualizing deities and seeing oneself travel ecstatically to the stars. The word for visualization is *cun*, which basically means "to be present" or "to exist." It is used here in its causative mode: "to cause to exist" or "to make present." It means that the meditator by an act of conscious concentration and focused intention causes certain energies to be present in the body and makes specific deities, scriptures, or travel scenes appear before the mind's eye.

While concentration creates control over the mind and insight practice effects a personality transformation, visualization makes the advanced Daoist into a full citizen of the otherworld, a god among the gods. Visualizing the deities as they come to reside in his or her human body, the adept is transformed into a replica of the cosmos, where the sun and the moon are the left and right eyes, the head is Mount Kunlun, and the ears are divine towers at the entrance to heaven. In this divine, cosmic form, Daoists then engage in ecstatic excursions to the otherworld, leaving their bodies behind and traveling widely in their spirits. They traverse the heavens, visit the palaces in the stars, and sojourn in the paradises of the immortals. They move freely about the far reaches of the earth and enter deep into the so-called grotto-heavens, passageways in the depth of the sacred mountains that connect to alternative universes, making the entire universe their true home (Robinet, *Taoist Meditation*).

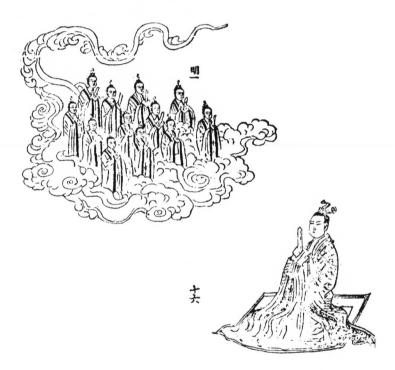

Fig. 38. Visualizing the arrival of celestial deities.

Doing so, they reach the ultimate state of cosmic identity, of oneness with the Dao and immortality in heaven. It can be described in terms of mystical union, a state of oneness with the deity and loss of individual self, commonly found in the mystical experience, which is described as ineffable, transient, felt to be true, and impossible to be consciously induced.

Mysticism also involves a religious quest that tends to proceed in three stages. Described by Evelyn Underhill in *Mysticism*, they are known as the purgative (emptying of old concepts), illuminative (gaining new insights), and unitive (attaining oneness or union) stages. They match the three levels of Daoist practice, the purification and reorientation of the body, the detached observation and transformation of emotions and the mind, and the attainment of oneness with the Dao either enstatically in oblivion or ecstatically through otherworldly journeys.

The worldview underlying Daoist meditation practice, moreover, closely corresponds to the concepts of other mystical traditions, described in theoretical discussions of mystical philosophy and presented especially in Aldous Huxley's *Perennial Philosophy*. This thinking makes four main points: (1) material reality is only the visible aspect of some deeper and more real ground; (2) human beings cannot perceive the ground with their senses but have the faculty to intuit it; (3) people as much as the world consist of two levels, a deep, real self and a superficial, desire-centered ego; (4) and the key to real life and truth is the shedding of the ego and recovery of the ground, both psychologically and in the world through mystical union.

Applied to Daoism, the ground is the Dao, which people participate in because they are born in this world but in their normal life and waking consciousness tend to ignore, reject, or leave behind. They cannot see or hear or touch it, but intuition, nonaction, and spontaneity will bring them closer to it. Both people and the world are suffused by the Dao, and there are practices that lead to a merging with it—physical, emotional, mental, and spiritual forms of cultivation. Individual identity is dissolved into the Dao and gives way to a larger and more cosmic existence, both here and in the otherworld.

Further Readings

Benson, Herbert. 1976. *The Relaxation Response*. New York: Avon.

Goleman, Daniel. 1988. *The Meditative Mind*. New York: George Putnam's Sons.

Hassan, Steven. 1988. *Combatting Cult Mind Control*. Rochester, VT: Park Street Press.

Huxley, Aldous. 1946. *The Perennial Philosophy*. London: Harper & Brothers.

Kohn, Livia. 1987. *Seven Steps to the Tao: Sima Chengzhen's Zuowanglun*. St.Augustin/Nettetal: Monumenta Serica Monograph XX.

_____, ed. 1989. *Taoist Meditation and Longevity Techniques*. Ann Arbor: University of Michigan, Center for Chinese Studies Publications.

_____. 1992. *Early Chinese Mysticism: Philosophy and Soteriology in the Taoist Tradition*. Princeton: Princeton University Press.

Lu, Kuan-yu. 1964. *The Secrets of Chinese Meditation*. London: Rider.

Robinet, Isabelle. 1993. *Taoist Meditation*. Translated by Norman Girardot and Julian Pas. Albany: State University of New York Press.

Roth, Harold D. 1999. *Original Tao: Inward Training and the Foundations of Taoist Mysticism*. New York: Columbia University Press.

Samuels, Mike, and Nancy Samuels. 1975. *Seeing with the Mind's Eye: The History, Technique, and Uses of Visualization*. New York: Random House.

Shapiro, Deane N., and Roger N. Walsh, eds. 1984. *Meditation: Classic and Contemporary Perspectives*. New York: Aldine.

Simonton, Oscar Carl. 1978. *Getting Well Again: A Step-by-Step, Self-Help Guide to Overcoming Cancer*. Los Angeles: J. P. Tardner.

Underhill, Evelyn. 1911. *Mysticism*. London: Methuen & Co.

Chapter 20

From Inner Alchemy to
Healing Dao

Daoist meditation is still practiced today in an integrated form known as inner alchemy (*neidan*). The dominant form of Daoist cultivation since the Song dynasty, it developed from earlier meditations under the influence of operative alchemy, replacing the physical materials of the cauldron with the internal energies of the body. Inner alchemy consists of a complex arrangement of techniques that integrates meditative longevity practices, operative alchemy, and the symbolism of the *Book of Changes*. Its goal is the attainment of immortality as a form of ecstatic otherworldly existence through a series of energetic bodily mutations, transforming the adept into a new spiritual entity at one with the Dao.

Reinventing the body in a new, mythological vision, practitioners identify seven treasures of immortality within. According to the twelfth-century *Wondrous Scripture of Daily Interior Practice* (*Nei riyong miaojing*), they are mercury (essence), gold (blood), jade (*qi*), crystal (marrow), agate (brain), nephrite (kidneys), and a central jewel (heart). To identify and transform these into pure spirit, adepts practice meditation while sitting quietly in a cross-legged position, preferably the lotus posture, with the spine erect and knees and buttocks firmly on the ground. The eyes are either closed or lowered, and the tongue is placed against the upper palate to facilitate the connection of the Governing and Conception Vessels. Men typically rest their hands in their lap, while women hold theirs up over the breasts. Other positions include reclining on one side with the head supported on a folded arm, standing in a steady pose, or walking slowly around—all still used in Qigong practice.

The meditation begins with an exercise in concentration, usually achieved by focusing on the breath as it enters and leaves the nostrils or on the rising and falling of the abdomen. This creates a focus of stillness and serenity in the body and gradually absorbs the practitioner to a point where all sensory impulses are ignored. As the *Wondrous Scripture of Daily Interior Practice* says:

213

First, sit alone in silent meditation,
Never allowing even a single thought to arise.
As the ten thousand affairs are all forgotten,
You can concentrate on spirit and firm up intention.
Keep the lips close to each other
And the teeth lightly touching.
Your eyes don't see a single thing,
Your ears don't hear a single sound.
Thus your mind is unified and focused within. (1a)

Similarly *Chongyang's Fifteen Articles on Establishing the Teaching* (*Chongyang lijiao shiwu lun*), a manual on early modern Daoist practice, says:

"Sitting straight" does not simply mean to sit with the body erect and eyes closed. That is superficial sitting. To truly sit you must maintain a mind like Mount Tai, unmovable and unshakable at all hours of the day, whether staying, walking, sitting, or lying down, in all forms of activity and repose.

Control and shut off the four gates of the senses — eyes, ears, mouth, and nose. Never let the outside world come in! If there is even a trace of a thought about activity and repose, this is no longer sitting quiet. If you can attain such a mind, although your body may remain in the world of dust, your name has already been entered in the ranks of the immortals. (sect. 2)

From this basis of stillness and sensory absorption, practitioners learn to see the world with the eyes of Dao, letting their Dao-nature shine forth instead of depending on personal evaluations and egotistic desires. Like the practitioners of inner observation, they overcome the ordinary mind and replace it increasingly the spirit.

Inner alchemy sees this transformation as a three-level process: from essence (*jing*) to energy (*qi*), from energy to spirit (*shen*), and from spirit to emptiness or the Dao. Practitioners begin by focusing on essence, the tangible form of *qi* that develops in the human body as it interacts with the world and appears most obviously as sexual energy — semen in men and menstrual blood in women. As described earlier in the discussion of sexual practices, adepts strive to control the outflow of *jing* and restore it to its original form as *qi*. After feeling the *jing* descend from the Ocean of *Qi*, men accordingly make it flow up along spine and into the head, thus "subduing the white tiger." Women, when they feel menstrual blood sink down from the Cavern of *Qi*, massage their breasts and visualize it rising upward and transforming into *qi*. Over several months, this will cause menstruation to cease, the "decapitation of the red dragon." Both then circulate the newly purified *qi* in the microcosmic orbit. Not only strengthening the body and enhancing health, this *qi*-circulation eventually leads to the manifestation of a concentrated pearl of primordial *qi* — newly formed in men, latently present from birth in women. The first stage concludes when the pearl coalesces.

The second stage is the same for men and women. It focuses on the transformation of purified *qi* into spirit. The pearl of dew is developed into the golden flower with the help of transmuted *qi*. For this, yin and yang are identified as different energies in the body, each described with different metaphors depending on the level of purity attained. Typically there are the following:

yang = heart = fire = trigram *li* ☲ = pure lead = dragon = red bird;
yin = kidneys = water = trigram *kan* ☵ = pure mercury = tiger = white tiger.

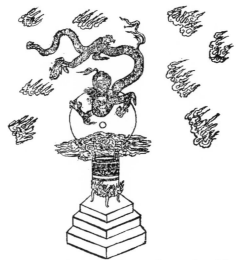

Fig. 39. The yang dragon plays with the pearl over the alchemical cauldron.

The texts describing these advanced practices tend to be rather obscure and highly metaphoric. An example is the long poem *Awakening to Perfection* (*Wuzhen pian*; trl. Cleary 1987) by the Daoist Zhang Boduan (984-1082). It says:

> In the crescent-moon furnace, jade blossoms grow;
> In the vermilion crucible, mercury flows evenly along.

Only after harmonizing them with great firing power
Can you plant the central pearl to gradually ripen. (Verse 4)

The lightning of true water boils and thunders in the realm of
metal and of water;
True fire arises from Mount Kunlun—these are our yin and
yang.
The two restored and harmonized in proper ways
Make the elixir grow naturally, pervade the body with its fra-
grance. (Verse 13)

Exercise: Reflect on the metaphors used for the interior agents and places of the body. Are they unique to China or do we find them in other cultures? How do they strike you? Do the images make sense? Can you find your own pictures for certain inner realities?

At each stage of the transmutation process, the energies are given different names and different metaphors are employed. Eventually adepts
learn not only to mix them in the abdomen but to revolve them through
an inner-body cycle that includes not only the spine and breastbone but
leads all the way to the feet and is known as the macrocosmic orbit.
Gradually one's energies are refined to a point where they become as
pure as the celestials themselves. Spirit emerges as an independent entity; the pearl opens up to give rise to the golden flower, the core of the
immortal embryo in the lower cinnabar field.

Once the embryo starts to grow, adepts switch their practice to nourish it
for ten months with embryo respiration. Not only nurturing the embryo,
this practice also makes the adept increasingly independent of outer
nourishment and air. While the first phase was easier for men, this stage
is easier for women because they are naturally endowed with the faculty
to grow an embryo. After ten months, the embryo is complete.

Adepts then proceed to the third stage. As Despeux and Kohn describe
in *Women in Daoism*, the as yet semi-material body of the embryo is transformed into the pure spirit body of the immortals, a body of primordial
qi. To attain its full realization, the embryo has to undergo several
phases. First it is nourished to completion and undergoes a spiritual
birth by moving up along the spine and exiting through the Hundred
Meeting (Baihui) point at the top of the head, which is now called Heavenly Gate (Tianguan). The first exiting of the spirit embryo is known as
"deliverance from the womb." It signifies the adept's celestial rebirth
and is accompanied by the perception of a deep inner rumbling, like a

clap of thunder. When the Heavenly Gate opens, a white smoky essence can be seen hovering above him or her. The spirit passes through the top of the head and begins to communicate with the celestials, thus transcending the limitations of the body.

Once the embryo has been born, it grows through a further meditative exercise known as "nursing for three years." Gradually getting used to its new powers, it moves faster and travels further afield until it can go far and wide without any limitation. As the spirit enters into its cosmic ventures, the adept exhibits supernatural powers, including the ability to be in two places at once, to move quickly from one place to another, to know past and future, to divine people's thoughts, and so on. Known as "spirit pervasion," this indicates the freedom achieved by the spirit as manifest in the practitioner. Eventually, the enlightenment gets strong and the adept, whose body is already transformed into pure light, overcomes life and death and melts into cosmic emptiness.

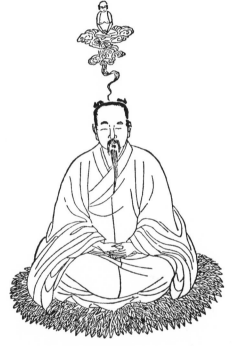

Fig. 40. The immortal embryo exits the body.

While it is possible to describe inner alchemy in terms of a well-structured and linear model, the tradition both encourages and rejects a straightforward understanding of the process. It makes heavy use of specific meditation techniques on various levels yet avoids seeing any particular method as the sole or even most direct path to deliverance. In its rejection of meditation as a systematic endeavor, inner alchemy follows the Chan Buddhist model, according to which sitting in meditation in order to attain enlightenment is like polishing a brick in order to make a mirror—impossible. The ultimate attainment is not something that results from any systematic, progressive practice but comes of itself. Prac-

tice just lays the foundation for events that occur on a completely different and more subtle plane. Much alchemical literature accordingly en-
gages in symbolic language and interprets both Buddhist and Daoist
concepts in a new and often unanticipated way.

In its modern adaptation, inner alchemy survives especially in the Healing Dao system, created by Mantak Chia. Originally from Thailand he
was born 1944. Recognized early for his spiritual potential, he began the
practice of Buddhist insight meditation at age six. During his teens, he
went to live in Hong Kong, where he learned Taiji quan, Aikido, and
Kundalini Yoga. There he met the Daoist master Yi Eng, who died at the
age of 168 and reportedly ate hardly any food for the last five years of his
life. From him Chia learned the practices of inner alchemy over five
years. Achieving expertise in these different methods, he decided to integrate them with Western thinking to enhance health, reduce stress, and
open higher spiritual awareness.

In 1978, Chia established a first Western foothold in Huntington, NY; in
1983, he opened a center in New York City. Today he resides in northern
Thailand but travels widely to give lectures and workshops. The main
Western teacher trained by Chia is Michael Winn, who founded the
Healing Dao University in upstate New York and supports local centers
that can be found in all metropolitan areas (www.healingdao.com).

The general theory of Healing Dao matches inner alchemy and Daoist
meditation. It sees the unfolding of spirituality in three levels:

1. create healing energy, strengthen and calm the body;
2. change negative emotions into strong, positive energy;
3. develop creative and spiritual practices.

On the first level, practitioners engage in Qigong and Taiji quan. They
begin their practice by shaking all parts of the body to loosen up and
release toxins. Then they practice deep breathing together with Qigong
standing meditations and qi-collecting techniques as well as a long and a
short form of Taiji quan. In all cases, muscles are consciously contracted
and relaxed to gain maximum flexibility and control. The pelvic area is
opened, and practitioners learn to tighten the perineum and feel the qi
move up along the spine. All this serves to open the body and strengthen
the qi-flow, greatly enhancing health and well-being.

For the second level, they move into several meditations that will clear
negative emotions, believed to be stored in the inner organs (Chia, *Iron*

Shirt Chi Kung, 145). Practices include the Inner Smile, the Six Healing Sounds, and the Microcosmic Orbit. The Inner Smile is best undertaken in a quiet place, a simple room, made comfortable with pillows and maybe with candles or incense. Practitioners dress comfortably and sit on the edge of a chair, their legs hip-distance apart, their feet flat on the floor. The back is straight, the head up, shoulders back and down, chin tucked in slightly. The hands rest comfortably in the lap, right palm on left. Close or lower the eyes and breathe normally.

The first step is to relax the forehead and envision a smiling energy flowing between the eyebrows to the nose and cheeks, allowing it to warm the whole face. Practitioners place the tongue on the roof of the mouth, to connect the Governing and Conception Vessels, and allow the jaw to release all tension. Taking the smiling feeling lower along the face, they smile into the neck and throat where a lot of stress accumulates and allow this area to open. Next, they smile into the throat area to the thyroid and parathyroid glands, which frees the ability to speak and communicate. From here, they let the *qi* flow down to the thymus gland, the seat of love and enlightenment, and allow it to moisten and grow bigger.

After this preparatory smiling, practitioners allow the *qi* to flow to the five inner organs in turn, envisioning them with their respective colors, appreciating them for their work, and allowing negative emotions to leave and positive virtues to enter. The practice concludes with the collection of smiling energy in the cinnabar field, where it is centered by being spiraled thirty-six times in an outward direction (women counterclockwise, men clockwise), then twenty-four times the other way.

> **Exercise:** Focus your attention on the area of your lungs. Feel them expand with inhalation and deflate with exhalation. Get a sense of fullness and strength in the lungs. Now envision a radiant white energy filling them. Let the lungs be rich and strong with the white energy. Smile at your lungs and develop a sense of appreciation for their continuous good work. Mentally thank them for their efforts and encourage them to be healthy and vigorous. Note that sadness and melancholy tend to manifest in the lungs. Let go of all sadness and melancholy, and instead invite in righteousness, the virtue associated with the lungs (www.healingdao.com; Chia and Chia, *Awaken Healing Light*).

The Inner Smile should be practiced daily, preferably upon waking up in the morning. An exercise of loving the body and appreciating its parts, its regular application energizes people and makes them more loving towards themselves and kinder towards others. It can also be practiced aiming at specific problems, and should be done more often in times of crisis, stress, anger, fear, or depression. By learning to smile into the tense part of the body until the tension melts and negative emotions become vital energy, people can express themselves more authentically. The organs, moreover, expand and become healthier as they feel appreciated and gain in relaxation and vitality.

The Six Healing Sounds were developed by Mantak Chia on the basis of the Six Breaths. They are similar to the Inner Smile in that practitioners begin by sitting with the spine erect and visualize the organs one by one, seeing them enwrapped in their respective colors. Then, while moving or stretching the arms in a particular way, they exhale with a hissing or rasping sound that causes the organ in question to vibrate at the correct frequency and supports the harmonizing of *qi*. Doing so, they release negative emotions from the organ while inviting positive virtues. The matching sounds, colors, emotions, and virtues are as follows:

Yin Organ	Yang Organ	Sound	Color	Emotion	Virtue
lungs	large intestine	sss	white	sadness	righteousness
kidneys	bladder	chooi	black	fear	compassion
liver	gallbladder	shhh	green	anger	benevolence
heart	small intestine	haw	red	excitement	sympathetic joy
spleen	stomach	ho	yellow	worry	wisdom
pericardium	triple heater	hsee			letting go

The Six Healing Sounds, too, should be practiced daily, preferably at bedtime or after other exercises. The practice facilitates heat exchange and detoxifies the organs (Chia and Chia, *Awaken Healing Light*).

The Microcosmic Orbit as practiced in Healing Dao also expands on traditional Daoist practice. It consists of making the *qi* flow up the Governing Vessel along the spine and down the Conception Vessel in the front of the torso. First, practitioners breathe repeatedly up and down the vessels to clear them. They start with a rather vigorous breath, then allow it to become smooth and quiet. Next, they breathe in a soft, easy circular flow to connect the two vessels, holding their tongue against the upper palate while inhaling up the spine and exhaling down the front. In a variation, they use the short sip method: six short, distinct in-breaths moving up the spine to the third eye, then six distinct out-breaths moving down the front.

The orbit can also be achieved without conscious breathing. Relaxing all breathing efforts, practitioners just engage in the visualization of *qi* as it flows up the spine and down the front. To enhance this, they may envision a golden tube filled with liquid flowing up and down the vessels or a bright fire or sun radiating up and down. To enhance the openness of the vessels a concentrated focus on specific energy points along either vessel can be applied, either mentally by maintaining concentration on the point and observing how it feels, or physically by massaging and palpitating a given area. The purpose of the practice is to open the body as much as possible to the free, smooth flow of *qi*, enhancing vital energy and creating the base for higher spiritual attainments (Chia and Chia, *Awaken Healing Light*).

The higher stages in Healing Dao involve the transformation of the self into a divine child and the creation of an inner sense of oneness with the Dao, an empowerment within the body that transcends the limitations of physical existence. This last stage is divided into five levels:

1. the birth of the immortal child through the absorption of higher forms of yin and yang, the sun and the moon, and by opening communication with the five spirit centers and the divinities of the four directions;

2. the maturation of the immortal child through feeding of the elixir of the sun, a series of meditations arranged according to one's astrological birth elements that involve the absorption of planetary power and ecstatic travels through the solar system;

3. the crystallization of the primordial spirit by focusing on the center in the head and there absorbing and interiorizing various astral forces, such as the Big Dipper, the Polestar, and the four Great Star quadrants, eventually attaining the ability to travel freely around them;

4. the merging of heaven and earth through opening a cosmic void within, where heaven and earth come together in primordial unity and where the physical body and personality of the adept fully dissolves into primordial *qi*;

5. union with the Dao, a spontaneous event that occurs when virtue, destiny, and cultivation are complete. (Winn, "Daoist Internal Alchemy," 28-30; Chia and Chia, *Iron Shirt Chi Kung*)

Although predominantly a spiritual practice, Healing Dao is also helpful for a host of medical conditions, including stress, tension, insomnia, constipation, dizziness, and others. Special techniques are also available for specific ailments. For the common cold, for example, adepts practice the microcosmic orbit while visualizing a warm fire moving through the vessels. They see the *qi* flowing through the nose and feel a sun warming the center of the body, radiating its revitalizing powers into the arms and legs. Fevers, on the other hand, require a cooling of the body, and adepts use the microcosmic orbit with the visualization of a cool, blue *qi* flowing along the channels. They ease pain with concentration and breathing exercises, opening the afflicted area and allowing *qi* to flow freely through it. Furthermore, they combat stress by focusing on the area of tension and releasing the emotions associated with it as well as by spiraling *qi* in the lower cinnabar field, creating a calming effect. Both inner alchemy and Healing Dao, therefore, continue classical Daoist meditation in their own way, paving the way for practitioners to attain of complete health, extend longevity, and the transcend to the immortals.

Further Readings

Chia, Mantak, and Maneewan Chia. 1986. *Iron Shirt Chi Kung*. New York: Healing Dao Center.

_____. 1993. *Awaken Healing Light of the Tao*. Huntington, NY: Healing Dao Books.

Cleary, Thomas. 1987. *Understanding Reality: A Taoist Alchemical Classic by Chang Po-tuan*. Honolulu: University of Hawai'i Press.

_____. 1992. *The Secret of the Golden Flower: The Classic Chinese Book of Life*. San Francisco: Harper.

Despeux, Catherine, and Livia Kohn. 2003. *Women in Daoism*. Cambridge, Mass.: Three Pines Press.

Lu Kuan-yü. 1970. *Taoist Yoga: Alchemy and Immortality*. London: Rider.

Ni, Hua-ching. 1992. *Internal Alchemy: The Natural Way to Immortality*. Santa Monica: College of Tao and Traditional Chinese Healing.

Skar, Lowell, and Fabrizio Pregadio. 2000. "Inner Alchemy (Neidan)." In *Daoism Handbook*, edited by Livia Kohn, 464-97. Leiden: E. Brill.

Winn, Michael. 2001. "Daoist Internal Alchemy: A Deep Language for Communicating with Nature's Intelligence." www.healingdao.com/cgi-bin/articles.pl

Conclusion

The Chinese tradition of health and long life has, over the millennia, brought forth a plethora of methods that have, ever since its earliest documentation in the ancient manuscripts, combined medical treatments with personal hygiene, life-enhancing techniques, and spiritual self-cultivation. Whether used singly or in conjunction with each other, they each contribute to greater integration of the human body-mind and lead to enhanced health and a higher sense of well-being. All the different methods have in common that they work with *qi*, the cosmic life-force that vitalizes the human body and is also at the root of the mind, society, and the natural world. Yet they also see the functioning of *qi* in slightly different ways and use different modalities to manipulate and adjust it.

The practice of acupuncture, moxibustion, and massage focuses on *qi* as a dynamic energy that flows in the meridians and is stored in the inner organs, able to move smoothly and steadily or give rise to excess and depletion. Practitioners stimulate *qi*-flow or release excess *qi* at specific acupuncture points or by manipulating the body's soft tissues, using the surface of the body to affect internal functions. Their view of *qi* is one of flow, like water, and many acupuncture points are known as "well," "river," or "ocean" points, acknowledging the water and channel vision of this mode of Chinese healing.

Unlike this, followers of herbs and diets see *qi* as the natural rising and falling, warming and cooling properties of the body. They modify it by adding, reducing, or eliminating substances in their daily intake, working primarily through the digestive tract rather than the meridian system, yet exerting an equally powerful impact on all aspects of the person. They understand *qi* less as a flowing energy than as an expanding and contracting cloud of vibrational particles. They apply food and herbs to heal by steadying the rhythm and frequency of these vibrations.

Yet another vision of *qi* inspires Fengshui, sexual techniques, and meditations that transform the emotions. Practitioners of these methods envision *qi* as fields or auras that develop in the individual and radiate outward, where they interact with other energy fields. These can be divided into natural and social fields, geomagnetic waves and human auras, environmental conditions and interpersonal relationships. The energy fields are seen as vibratory systems that can either entrain or clash with each other, creating harmony or increasing discord. Health is consequently a function of vibrational harmony in the interactive energy fields, since nobody escapes the impact of nature and other people. Efforts at living in a *qi*-rich environment, creating a harmonious constellation of rooms and furniture thus go hand in hand with the establishment of joyful and positive relationships. Sexual intercourse, then, the most intimate and potent form of energy exchange, needs particular attention, since it can lead to massive *qi*-depletion or the attainment of highest bliss.

Adepts of Chinese self-cultivation, finally, often inspired by Daoism, view *qi* as a cosmic, spiritual potency and work with it on the subtle level of *shen* or spirit. They emphasize the need to focus intention, the carrier of *shen*, on the specific body part that is being activated—be it through breathing, meditation, or slow movements. Their goal is to vitalize the entire person with the subtlest form of *qi*, creating wholeness and enhancing a sense of connectedness to the larger universe. People following these practices may begin with the goal of attaining health, but they soon find other effects, such as a heightened sensitivity, a greater appreciation of nature and life, and a feeling of peace and harmony. Breathing consciously and moving in relation to heaven and earth, they begin to transcend the limitations of the body and find themselves entrained with the subtle vibrations of the cosmos.

Qi, although essentially only one fundamental cosmic energy, can thus be understood and applied in all these different ways: as a water-like flow through the meridians, as vibratory particles that warm and cool the body, as energy fields in close interaction with outside entities, and as spiritual potency in harmony with the Dao. However one prefers to think of it and whichever modality one chooses to access it, one's actions, whether positive or negative, have a pervasive impact on the entire body-mind and, by extension, on the social life and good fortune of the individual. They influence the entirety of being—self, society, and cosmos.

As the Chinese way to health and long life presents a complete and integrated network of different *qi*-visions and healing methods, it is not surprising that many people have positive experiences with Chinese practices and find themselves increasingly drawn to them. Also, while the dominant medical establishment is still characterized by an "enduring and widespread academic skepticism and myopia about therapeutic approaches that are based on concepts of energy" (Oschman, *Energy Medicine*, 1), research in biology, physiology, and physics has opened up many new venues of looking at energy healing. These branches of science are beginning to create a language that will eventually allow Western science to account for the Chinese concepts of body-mind and health, demystify the phenomenon and experiences of *qi*, and make them more widely accessible to the general public.

The most important new concepts emerging from this research are measurable biomagnetic fields and bioelectricity. Biomagnetic fields are human energy centers that vibrate at different frequencies, storing and giving off energies not unlike the inner organs in the Chinese system. Their energetic output or vibrations can be measured, and it has been shown that the heart and the brain continuously pulse at extremely low frequencies (ELF). It has also become clear through controlled measurements that biomagnetic fields are unbounded so that, for example, the field of the heart vibrates beyond the body and extends infinitely into space, verifying the Chinese conviction that people and the universe interact continuously on an energetic level.

Similarly, bioelectricity manifests in energy currents that crisscross the human body and are similar to the meridians of acupuncture. Separate from and, in evolutionary terms, more ancient than the nervous system, these currents work through the so-called cytoskeleton, a complex net of connective tissue that is a continuous and dynamic molecular webwork. Also known as the "living matrix," this webwork contains so-called integrins or trans-membrane linking molecules which have no boundaries but are intricately interconnected. When touching the skin or inserting an acupuncture needle, the integrins make contact with all parts of the body through the matrix webwork. Based on this evidence, wholeness is becoming an accepted concept, which sees "the body as an integrated, coordinated, successful system" and accepts that "no parts or properties are uncorrelated but all are demonstrably linked" (Oschman, *Energy Medicine*, 49, citing E. F. Adolph).

Mental and emotional states are accordingly integrated into the larger picture, and intention is seen as a kind of directed vibration that can have a disturbing or enhancing effect on health. Mental attitudes give rise to specific patterns of energy so that magnetic activity in the nervous system of the individual can spread through his or her body into the energy fields and bodies of others. This understanding accounts for the efficacy of therapeutic touch and distant energy healing, during which the practitioner goes into a meditative state of mind and directs healing thoughts toward the patient. Measuring experiments have shown that the field emanating from the hands of a skilled practitioner is very strong, sometimes reaching a million times the strength of the normal brain field. It can, moreover, contain infrared radiation, creating heat and spreading light as part of the healing effort (see Gerber, *Vibrational Medicine*).

The living matrix is simultaneously a mechanical, vibrational, energetic, electronic, photonic, and informational network. It consists of a complex, linked pattern of pathways and molecules that forms a tensegrity system. A term taken originally from architecture where it is used in the structural description of domes, tents, sailing vessels, and cranes, tensegrity indicates a continuous tensional network (tendons) connected by a set of discontinuous elements (struts), which can also be fruitfully applied to the description of the wholeness of the body.

> The body as a whole, and the spine in particular, can usefully be described as tensegrity systems. In the body, bones act as discontinuous compression elements and the muscles, tendons and ligaments act as a continuous tensional system. Together the bones and tensional elements permit the body to change shape, move about, and lift objects. (Oschman, *Energy Medicine*, 153)

This understanding of the body as a tensegrity system allows for the analysis of physical and movement therapies, such as *daoyin*, Qigong, and Taiji quan as well as the Western methods of Feldenkrais, Alexander, and structural integration (Rolfing). It is becoming evident that bodily posture and modes of movement are essential to the way people feel and act. Straighter posture and better balance allow bioelectric energies to flow more freely, improve the ability of the body to adapt to changing situations (plasticity), and enhance the efficiency of the body's use. Also, correct movements may contribute to the release of traumas and tensions stored in the joints and muscles of the body, providing access to greater health and well-being.

Health can also be enhanced with the use of crystals in healing which correspond to the inherently crystalline nature of living tissues." Living crystals, composed of long, thin, pliable molecules," are found in the body "in arrays of phospholipid molecules forming cell membranes and myelin sheaths of nerves, collagen arrays forming connective tissue and fascia, contractile arrays in muscle, arrays of sensory elements in the eye, nose, and ear, arrays of microtubules, microfilaments, and other fibrous components of the cytoskeleton" (Oschman, *Energy Medicine*, 129). All these different aspects of the body can be enhanced and regulated with the help of natural crystals, such as quartz, shells, and certain stones, since crystalline objects resonate powerfully with each other, setting up electromagnetic fields that support and enhance each other.

The power of crystals and their vibratory resonance is already used technologically in modern medicine in so-called PEMF, or "pulsed electromagnetic field" therapy. A battery-powered pulse generator connects to a coil that is placed next to a patient's injury, especially in cases when the area has stopped improving after a trauma. Radiating healing pulses toward the injured body part for several hours every day, this produces a magnetic field in the body, inducing currents to flow again and thereby jump-starting the healing process. It is especially useful in healing bones after fractures but can also be applied to other injuries (Oschman, *Energy Medicine*, 73).

These experiences and various related experiments in the scientific community are gradually making energy healing an approachable and understandable mode of medicine. While still far removed from the common mainstream, they are establishing a bridge between Chinese and other traditional forms of healing and modern Western science. As the quantum model of the universe sinks deeper into scientific consciousness and measuring apparatuses grow subtler and more sophisticated, all those phenomena now associated with quackery and extrasensory perception will more and more move into the sphere of the known and become acceptable and even inevitable parts of medical science. The Chinese way of health and long life, increasingly translated into the new language of energy healing, will finally come to play its rightful role in the great endeavor of human fulfillment.

Further Readings

Becker, Robert O., and Gary Sheldon. 1985. *The Body Electric: Electromagnetism and the Foundation of Life*. New York: William Morrow and Co.

Bentov, Itchak. 1977. *Stalking the Wild Pendulum: On the Mechanics of Consciousness*. New York: E. P. Dutton.

Gerber, Richard. 1988. *Vibrational Medicine: New Choices for Healing Ourselves*. Santa Fe: Bear and Company.

Oschman, James. 2000. *Energy Medicine: The Scientific Basis*. New York: Churchill Livingstone.

Zohar, Dana. 1990. *The Quantum Self*. New York: William Morrow.

Index

Other Titles from Three Pines Press

Cosmos and Community: The Ethical Dimension of Daoism
A full-length treatment of Daoist ethics based on new translations from primary sources, this examines Daoist rules in three types of community: lay organizations, monastic institutions, and the closed communities of millenarian or utopian groups. The book follows four major kinds of rules—prohibitions, admonitions, concrete injunctions, and personal resolutions—then discusses the sources and translates original texts. Further translations are available as an electronic publication: "Supplement to *Cosmos and Community*." $29.95

Daoism and Chinese Culture
A proven textbook for use in introductory classes on Daoism, Chinese religion, history, and culture, this work presents a chronological survey thematically divided into four parts: Ancient Thought, Religious Communities, Spiritual Practices, and Modernity. The book makes ample use of original materials and provides references to further readings and original sources in translation. $19.95

Women in Daoism
Divided into three parts—"Goddesses," "Immortals and Priestesses," and "Women's Transformation"—this cooperative work details the historical development and general role of women in the Daoist tradition, focusing on the different ideals women stood for, their positions as nuns and priestesses, and their specific religious practices. $25.00

Title Index to Daoist Collections
A combined and standardized index for all collections of Daoist texts this presents separate title indexes to the seven Daoist collections, followed by an alphabetical index to all titles. Easy to use, it gives access to all Daoist texts collected over the centuries and provides a clear, standarized way of referring to them. $45.00

Electronic Publications from Three Pines Press

Chen Tuan: Discussions and Translations

Based on the author's dissertation on Chen Tuan (Frankfurt: Peter Lang, 1981) and on several articles, this presents three discussion essays on Chen Tuan as an immortal and his role in the legitimation of the Song dynasty, plus six translations of both biographical and religious materials.

Living With the Dao: Conceptual Issues in Daoist Practice

This collection brings together ten essays that address key issues relevant to Daoist practice, such as concepts of evil, the relation of body and mind, stages of Qigong practice. Based on careful reading of medieval Daoist texts, the papers show a keen awareness of practitioners' perspectives.

Supplement to 'Cosmos and Community'

Translations of an fifteen important religious texts, covering the entire Daoist tradition, from the early Celestial Masters to seventeenth-century Complete Perfection. A valuable resource for the study of ethics and community organization.

$10.00 each, no S&H

www.threepinespress .com

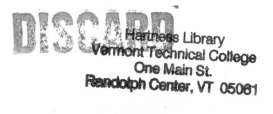